# Pressure Sore

# Pre          on

# Pressure Sore Prevention

**Alison Simpson, RGN, PG Dip.**
Nursing Practice Development Adviser
Chelsea & Westminster Healthcare NHS Trust, London

**Kate Bowers, BA (Hons), RGN**
Nursing Research Development Adviser
Chelsea & Westminster Healthcare NHS Trust, London

**Dickon Weir-Hughes, MA, RGN, MRSH**
Assistant Director of Nursing
Chelsea & Westminster Healthcare NHS Trust, London

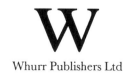

Whurr Publishers Ltd

© 1996 Whurr Publishers Ltd
First published 1996 by
Whurr Publishers Ltd
19b Compton Terrace, London N1 2UN, England

Reprinted 1997

**British Library Cataloguing in Publication Data**
A catalogue record for this book is available from the
British Library.

ISBN 1-86156 010 9

Printed and bound in the UK by Athenaeum Press Ltd,
Gateshead, Tyne & Wear

# Contents

# Acknowledgements

This book was originally developed as part of the Pressure Sore Prevention Strategy for Chelsea & Westminster Healthcare NHS Trust, London. The authors wish to acknowledge the assistance provided by multidisciplinary professionals throughout the organisation, whose expertise and firm commitment have been fundamental and enormously valuable.

# Foreword

Pressure sores are not a new phenomenon, however they represent an ongoing challenge to healthcare providers. It is considered that pressure sores are largely preventable and a reduction in their prevalence must therefore be a matter of priority for any healthcare provider. Furthermore, healthcare is offered in an increasingly competitive market, and pressure sore prevalence data are considered by purchasers of healthcare services to be a key indicator of the quality of care provided.

Pressure sores have a complex and multifactorial aetiology and, in tackling this challenge, it is therefore essential for healthcare providers to have a considered and comprehensive strategy for their prevention, which defines and promotes optimum standards of preventative practice. The development and implementation of such a strategy requires the involvement and commitment of all staff at all levels within a healthcare provider unit.

This book has been adapted from a strategy document developed and implemented by Chelsea & Westminster Healthcare NHS Trust. The strategy document was developed by reviewing the vast quantity of literature that has been generated on this subject and with the collaboration of a large number of professionals and other staff working within the Trust. As a result the Trust has significantly reduced the prevalence of pressure sores and, in this light, I would recommend this book to be used as a base from which others can develop their own strategies.

Sarah E Mullally, RGN, BSc (Hons) Nursing, MSc.
Director of Nursing and Quality
Chelsea & Westminster Healthcare NHS Trust

# Chapter 1:
# Introduction

The purpose of this book is to define and guide good practice and to support decision making in the prevention of pressure sores. It has been developed largely by reviewing the literature that has been generated on this subject.

## The Problem

Pressure sores are not a new phenomenon. From the beginning of recorded history pressure sores have been reported as one of the most constant problems plaguing the disabled, debilitated and chronically ill, and early investigators developed a good understanding of the aetiology of pressure sores (Torrance, 1983). Considerable work has been undertaken on the subject of pressure sores, particularly over the past 30 years, and today there is a large volume of literature on this so-called worldwide 'epidemic'. Yet, despite this progress in the understanding of the aetiology and prevention of pressure sores, they remain a challenge. It is therefore suggested that this knowledge has been underutilised.

In 1992 the Department of Health estimated that 6.7% of the adult hospital population were affected by pressure sores. It has been suggested that most pressures sores (up to 95%) are preventable if there is early prediction of an individual's susceptibility and an active prevention programme is implemented. This claim is well documented in the literature (for example Hibbs, 1988; Waterlow, 1988b).

## Whose Problem?

There are two pervading beliefs concerning pressure sores that arguably impede optimal prevention. They are both related to 'ownership' of the problem.

1

The first is the widely held view that pressure sores are a nursing problem. This is an unfortunate view because, in practice, it has led to an implied, but erroneous, belief that pressure sore formation equates to poor nursing care. Indeed, for many years nurses have carried the burden of guilt in relation to the occurrence of pressure sores (Dealey, 1992a). This belief has led to a lack of multidisciplinary team collaboration and accountability for the prevention of pressure sores. It is now well recognised that pressure sores have a complex and multifactorial aetiology, and to attribute their occurrence to poor nursing care only demonstrates a failure to appreciate this fact. However, this uniprofessional nursing perspective of pressure sores is now considered to be changing (Sutton and Wallace, 1990). The need for a multidisciplinary team approach is increasingly recognised in the effective prevention of pressure sores.

The second popularly held belief is that pressure sores are a problem exclusive to the elderly population; the implication being that they are an expected problem within departments of medicine for the elderly (Young and Dobrzanski, 1992). There are several reasons why this view cannot be sustained. Although it has been suggested that approximately 70% of pressure sores occur in individuals over 70 years of age (Young and Dobrzanski, 1992), many larger scale studies have identified younger groups of individuals at risk (Barbenal et al., 1977; Bliss, 1988; Reuler and Cooney, 1981). Recent demographic trends indicate an increasing elderly proportion of the population, which accounts for the fact that elderly individuals are no longer exclusively admitted to departments of elderly medicine, but that they now comprise the largest group under treatment in most hospital wards and departments. Moreover, improved primary care and community support increasingly enable sick elderly individuals to be cared for at home. The necessary expertise and equipment for pressure sore prevention management therefore also need to be available in the community.

It is now recognised that pressure sore prevention strategies require not a fragmented and disjointed approach but a centrally planned and coordinated strategy (King's Fund Centre, 1989).

## Cost to the Individual

For the individual a pressure sore can cause pain, misery, systemic illness, increased length of stay in hospital, extended absence from work and normal activities, loss of earnings, reduced self-esteem, altered body image and may sufficiently delay rehabilitation measures to preclude return to independence (Hibbs, 1988).

### Mortality

The mortality directly ascribable to pressure sores is difficult to determine, because for many individuals the underlying medical condition(s) is life threatening in its own right. There is no doubt however that pressure sores are accompanied by increased mortality. The relative mortality risk for elderly individuals with pressure sores in one study was found to be fivefold higher than for similar elderly people without pressure sores (Norton, 1962). One report, referring to Office of Population Census and Surveys statistics, states that 'nationally, in 1986, 171 death certificates recorded pressure sores as a cause of death, with 1,929 mentions' (Davies et al., 1991). It suggests that this may represent only the tip of the proverbial iceberg and that, because of professional defensiveness, mortality from pressure sores may be considerably under-reported.

## Cost to the National Health Service (NHS)

For the NHS, patients with chronic wounds are expensive in terms of human and other resources (Hibbs, 1988: Livesley, 1987). The total cost of hospital care for one patient with a severe pressure sore in 1988 was calculated to be in excess of £25,000 (Hibbs, 1988). Extended hospital stays also result in lost opportunities to treat other cases, to which it is difficult to apportion costs. The true cost of pressure sores is unknown. Cost estimates have ranged from £60 million to £200 million a year (Department of Health, 1993b). To help clarify this, the Department of Health commissioned Touche Ross to report on the cost of pressure sores to the health NHS (Department of Health, 1993b). The report looked at the relative cost and the financial trade-off between treatment of pressure sores and an effective pressure sore prevention policy. The report was solely concerned with the costs to the NHS, i.e. it excluded quality of life costs to the individual. Touche Ross concluded that the financial cost of preventing pressures sores in a hospital may be similar to the cost of treating pressure sores, and indicated that the identification of individuals at risk of developing pressure sores is therefore very important in determining the cost of implementing prevention plans. In other words, the cost of prevention may be more expensive than treatment if a larger number of individuals receive preventative interventions than would develop a sore and require treatment.

The key to cost-effective prevention is therefore accurate and ongoing individual risk assessment in order that resources are effectively targeted. Cost savings from effective prevention strategies may also lie in saved opportunity costs resulting from shorter lengths of stay rather than 'cash in hand'. Touche Ross also stated that it should be borne in mind that a small number of successful cases of litigation can dramatically alter the cost/saving ratio. They also stated that, on ethical grounds, pressure sores should always be avoided wherever practicable, because of the advantageous outcomes in terms of health gain and quality of life. The burden of successful litigation considerably adds to the financial cost of pressure sores. Some patients and their families have been awarded damages in excess of £100,000 (cited in Robertson, 1987).

The healthcare services of NHS Trust hospitals are offered in an increasingly competitive market. Pressure sore prevalence and incidence data are considered to be key indicators of the quality of care provided within a hospital (Audit Commission, 1991).

## Summary points

- In 1992 the Department of Health estimated that 6.7% of the adult hospital population were affected by pressure sores
- Literature suggests that most pressure sores (95%) are preventable (Hibbs, 1988; Waterlow, 1988b)
- Pressure sores have a complex and multifactorial aetiology — the multidisciplinary team share the responsibility of this problem
- Pressure sores can affect individuals of any age in all hospital wards and departments (Barbenal et al., 1977; Bliss, 1988; Reuler and Cooney, 1981)
- For the individual, a pressure sore can cause pain, misery, systemic illness, increased length of stay in hospital, extended absence from work and normal activities, loss of earnings, reduced self-esteem, altered body image and may sufficiently delay active rehabilitation measures to preclude return to independence (Hibbs, 1988)
- Healthcare purchasers consider pressure sore prevalence and incidence data to be key indicators of the quality of care delivered in a provider unit (Audit Commission, 1991)

- It is difficult to establish the true cost of pressure sores to the NHS. It has been estimated that the cost is in excess of £60 million per year (Department of Health, 1993b)
- Damages in excess of £100,000 have been awarded for the development of a pressure sore in hospital (cited in Robertson, 1987)

# Chapter 2:
# Legal Issues

There is good reason to believe that patients are becoming increasingly concerned about pressure sores as an unnecessary and preventable complication of hospital treatment, and are beginning to seek recompense through the courts. Damages in excess of £100,000 have already been awarded to a successful claimant (the case of Silver cited in Robertson, 1987).

As healthcare professionals, we have a legal duty of care for our patients. Patients have the right to expect healthcare professionals to care for them in the most effective manner. This raises the questions 'can the development of pressure sores in a patient be considered as a failure by the healthcare professionals concerned to execute their duty of care?' and 'are we therefore legally culpable?' The questions are really those of negligence. A patient might well argue that the pain and suffering of a pressure sore were the result of negligent care, and seek compensation from the healthcare organisation concerned. In such a case, the burden would be on the patient (the plaintiff) to prove that:

- the healthcare professionals concerned had a legal duty of care;
- there was a breach in that duty of care;
- the patient suffered damage or injury as a direct result of that breach in duty of care.

There would be little difficulty in establishing that the healthcare professionals concerned had a legal duty of care. There would be a breach in that duty of care if the healthcare professionals concerned failed to make every reasonable effort to prevent the pressure sore from developing where this was possible. Assuming that the patient was not immobilised for a long period of time prior to hospital admission then, given the literature available, the patient would have little difficulty in establishing that preventative action was practicable. Having established this, evidence would then have to be produced to demonstrate that the healthcare professionals had failed to take appropriate action. The court would seek to establish what would have been 'reasonable care' in the circumstances. Evidence of assessment of risk and appropriate care planning would be sought. Ignorance of appropriate care derived from valid and reliable research would not be an adequate defence, because a patient has a legal right to expect such from competent healthcare professionals. Healthcare professionals are also required by their regulatory bodies to maintain and improve their knowledge and competence. Witnesses would be called to testify that the patient had, or had not, received care as planned. Patient records would also be reviewed. Evidence of continued evaluation of the care planned would be sought. Seeking testimony to the presence of a pressure sore would pose few problems.

Most people accept that individual practitioners are responsible and can be held to account for their actions. But pressure sores are most likely to arise not from actions, but from a failure to act. This distinction should not allow healthcare professionals to think that they are less responsible for having omitted to take action to promote and safeguard a patient than for having acted directly to harm the patient. Whilst an employer will normally accept vicarious liability for personnel working in the course of their employment, he or she may take disciplinary action against an employee whose actions were found to contradict his or her expectations for standards of practice, as determined in policies, procedures and professional guidelines. In addition, a healthcare professional involved in any legal proceedings may also be found guilty of misconduct by his or her professional regulatory body.

The very real threat of litigation, in addition to inquiry from their regulatory body and their employer, might lead some healthcare professionals to reassess their priorities. However, defensive practice will not benefit patients in the long-term and ethical, rather than legal, justification for high-quality care should be more persuasive and fundamental to those working in the healthcare professions. There will undoubtedly be cases in which previous care or the patient's debilitated condition impedes the effectiveness of preventative action. However, the duties to promote health and healing and to prevent harm and complications from ill health are values so fundamental to healthcare professionals that to omit consideration for pressure sore prevention amounts to unethical practice.

## Summary points

- Pressure sore development in hospital can lead to large claims for compensation
- Healthcare professionals have a legal duty of care for their patients
- Liability can arise from a failure to make every reasonable effort to prevent pressure sores developing where this is possible
- Defensive practice is not beneficial to patients — ethical rather than legal justification for high-quality care should be more persuasive and fundamental to those working in the healthcare professions
- Pressure sore prevention must be based on accepted research evidence
- A causal link must be established between care inadequacies and the damage or injury claimed by the patient
- Patient records are very important in providing evidence of appropriate patient assessment, care planning, care delivery and evaluation of care

# Chapter 3:
# Nursing
# Documentation

The United Kingdom Central Council for Nursing, Midwifery and Health Visiting (UKCC) 'Code of Professional Conduct' (1992) states that all registered nurses, midwives and health visitors are personally accountable for their own practice and, in exercising their professional accountability must:
'ensure that no action or omission on their part, or within their sphere of responsibility, is detrimental to the interests, condition or safety of patients or clients'.

Documentation is an important way of exercising accountability in the prevention of pressure sores. Effective documentation provides healthcare professionals with an opportunity to record actions and in-actions and provides others with information on when, where, why, what and how specific conditions occurred. Nursing documentation is therefore the major medium through which nurses demonstrate their legal, professional and public accountability.

## Record of Patient Assessment

The nursing assessment of a patient forms the basis on which nursing intervention is planned, and as such should provide accurate, current and comprehensive information concerning the patient's condition. It is recommended that an individual's pressure sore risk status should be documented within 12 hours of admission to hospital or other healthcare setting, and then at appropriate intervals as dictated by the overall state of the patient's health.

Risk assessment tools should be used as they provide the basis of a systematic approach to the assessment of risk of pressure sore development. Further information about risk assessment tools can be found in chapter 7. Which risk assessment tool to use is largely a matter for personal preference, provided the user is aware of the tool's strengths and limitations. However, the tools should be used as an adjunct to, rather than the basis of, the nursing assessment. Risk factors specific to the individual patient will require a more detailed assessment.

## Reassessment of Risk Status

Reassessment of an individual's risk status is particularly important in the initial period of his or her hospital admission. Norton (1962) reported that of some 250 patients admitted to a geriatric hospital and assessed using the Norton score, many of these patients' scores fell during the first 2 weeks of admission and this was accompanied by subsequent pressure sore development (cited in Flanagan, 1993). Patients who experience significant health changes while in hospital will require frequent reassessment so that the care plan can be appropriately adjusted. It is recommended that the minimum standard for the frequency of risk assessment is weekly.

## Record of Skin Pressure Damage

Chapter 11 of this book describes a recently developed 4-stage pressure sore classification system. Whilst the use of such a classification system for audit purposes represents good practice, its use within nursing documentation is limited. Pressure damage graded at stage 2 or above will require more comprehensive documentation than is provided by the classification system. For example, characteristics of the sore(s) such as its dimensions, other clinical indicators and the individual's experience of the sore(s) will require concise and clear documentation. Wound assessment charts provide a useful assessment framework. Where possible, measurements of pressure-damaged skin should be taken. Methods of measurement include using a clean paper ruler, or wound tracing using, for example, a transparent plastic wound mapping grid (for example, the 3M mapping chart), or a clean latex glove. However, measurements of three-dimensional wounds require alternative techniques such as depth gauges and installations with normal saline to gauge the volume of wound cavity (McTaggart, 1994). Photographs also serve to provide a record of the appearance of skin pressure damage.

Pressure-related erythema may be considered to be the normal response of healthy tissue to sustained pressure, or else indicative of underlying skin damage, that is it may be either blanching or non-blanching (see chapter 6). Erythema that blanches on the application of finger pressure may be considered as grade 0 pressure damage, whereas grade 1 pressure damage is characterised by non-blanching erythema. Accurate assessment of pressure-related erythema is therefore critical and should be clearly documented.

## Plans of Care

The UKCC's document 'Standards for Records and Record Keeping' (1993) states that, where possible, records should be written in terms that the patient or client will be able to understand, and as such aid service user involvement in the implementation and provision of care. Plans of care formulated by first-level registered nurses, in relation to the prevention or management of pressure sores, must be patient-focused and include patient education where appropriate. Plans of care should reflect a multidisciplinary approach to the prevention and management of pressure sores by including the contributions of non-nursing healthcare professionals.

## Evaluations and the Use of Abbreviations

The purpose of written evaluations is to establish the efficacy of nursing and other healthcare professionals' interventions, by documenting the patient's response to care and treatment. Evaluation records also act as an essential means of communication for those members of the healthcare team providing such care and treatment. It is important therefore that such evaluations are made as soon as possible after the events to which they relate, and are accurate, concise and comprehensive. Abbreviations and meaningless phrases, for example, '2 hourly PAC', should not appear within nursing documentation.

## Summary points

- Nursing documentation is a major medium through which nurses demonstrate their accountability
- Risk assessment tools should be used only as a component of a more comprehensive individual nursing assessment
- Reassessment of individual risk in relation to pressure sore development is particularly important during the initial period of hospital admission and/or in the event of significant health changes being experienced by the patient
- The written record of skin pressure damage should be an

informative one that incorporates methods of wound measurement where appropriate

- Skin erythema should be documented as either blanching (grade 0), or non-blanching (grade 1)
- Plans of care should be written in such a way that where possible patients may be informed and involved in the care that they receive
- Abbreviations and phrases that fail to provide real meaning should not be used in any nursing documentation

# Chapter 4:
# Professional Roles

A wide range of professionals are involved in the prevention of pressure sores. It is generally accepted that only through effective multidisciplinary collaboration can the prevalence of pressure sores be successfully reduced. This chapter aims to outline the responsibilities of each professional group involved. Many ancillary services also contribute to effective pressure sore prevention. The responsibilities of these services are also indicated. All professionals are responsible for maintaining and updating their knowledge in relation to pressure sore prevention.

## Hospital Directors and Professional Leaders

Hospital directors and professional leaders have overall responsibility in facilitating good quality of care through the appropriate targeting of resources and the provision of educational support to staff. They must ensure that appropriate systems of work are in place to facilitate the process of pressure sore prevention. This will include ensuring that such systems are effective, using the audit process, and that suitable equipment is available.

## Doctors

In many environments the doctor will have overall responsibility to plan and coordinate patient medical treatments. Specifically, doctors have responsibility to maintain the patient's optimum physiological condition, with particular reference to hydration, nutrition, respiratory function, circulation and infection during treatment. Where appropriate, they should also ensure referral to other professional disciplines in order to employ their specialist knowledge in assessing the need for and planning of appropriate care interventions.

# Nurses

Registered nurses have prime responsibility for ensuring that an holistic approach is maintained in the management of patient care. They should identify those patients at risk of developing pressure sores by considering known predisposing and precipitating factors, and then plan, implement and evaluate appropriate research-based care. They also have a coordinating role for the whole multidisciplinary team. Registered nurses are responsible for the selection of suitable equipment and for ensuring that equipment employed in pressure sore prevention is in good working order and protected from potentially preventable damage. Registered nurses are accountable for the nursing care that their patients receive and should therefore ensure that nursing students and healthcare assistants are appropriately supervised in care delivery. They also have an important role in educating students, healthcare assistants, other professionals, patients and their carers.

# Healthcare Assistants

Healthcare assistants have an important role in supporting and complementing professional nursing practice by allowing registered nurses to use their skills and time appropriately in the areas for which they are uniquely qualified (Royal College of Nursing, 1993). Healthcare assistants are responsible for ensuring that certain aspects of care are implemented in accordance with the care plan prescribed by the registered nurse and for reporting to the registered nurse any changes in the condition of the patient's pressure areas.

# Dieticians

Dieticians are responsible for making detailed nutritional assessments of patients referred to them and identifying which particular nutrients may be insufficient in the patient's diet to provide the necessary conditions for maintaining skin integrity. The dietician will provide advice and will plan and arrange where necessary an appropriate diet. In addition, the dietician will monitor and review the patient's progress. Dieticians and nurses should work closely together to ensure that the patient is optimally nourished.

# Occupational Therapist

The occupational therapist is available to assess a patient's functional abilities, and to recommend and advise on any problems that a patient has in performing those activities of daily living which contribute to the risk of pressure sore formation. They will advise on the suitability and correct use of specialist equipment, such as cushions, seating, wheelchairs and cutlery.

## Physiotherapist

The physiotherapist has a dual role. Firstly, in providing care interventions that promote a variety of suitable positions and techniques to improve the patient's voluntary movement and independence. When the patient has no voluntary movement, or is unable to transfer weight in any way, this must be subsidised by a member of staff. Secondly, the physiotherapist has an important role in teaching other professionals to handle and position patients so as to minimise trauma to the skin and promote recovery.

## Portering Staff

Portering staff have an important role in ensuring that patients are transferred within the hospital in a timely manner. Portering staff may also have responsibility for the prompt delivery of specialist pressure-relieving devices to wards and departments in some hospitals. They have responsibility to protect this equipment from damage whilst in transit between wards and departments.

## Bioengineers

Bioengineers have a responsibility to evaluate and maintain the performance of equipment employed in pressure sore prevention.

## Equipment Suppliers

Equipment suppliers have a responsibility to ensure that orders receive prompt attention and that goods are delivered in a timely manner. When equipment is on loan they are responsible for ensuring that effective strategies are in place for equipment monitoring, maintenance and replacement. They are also responsible for ensuring that equipment users possess the knowledge required to optimise its benefits to the patient.

## Patients

Patients are responsible for furthering their own health gain and avoiding further deterioration of their health to the best of their knowledge, capability and motivation at the time. Patients are often dependent on the multidisciplinary team to provide them with information related to their condition and practical ways of helping themselves. Further information can be found in chapter 10 on education.

## Action Points

When a patient is identified as being at risk of developing pressure sores, the following actions should be pursued:

- Liaison with other members of the multidisciplinary team as appropriate — in all cases the doctor responsible for the patient's treatment should be alerted
- Communication with other departments to which the patient may be transferred or visit
- Information concerning pressure sore prevention is discussed with the patient and relatives, where appropriate
- Where a patient at risk of developing pressure sores is being discharged into the community, early liaison must take place in order that special provision for continuation of appropriate preventative care can be made. In some cases the district nurse may visit the patient prior to discharge in order to make a needs assessment
- In the same way, where a patient at risk of developing pressure sores is transferred from the community in to hospital, the district nurse will liaise with the hospital ward or department concerned
- All patients who are transferred within the hospital or discharged from hospital must have the following in their records:
  - Evidence of comprehensive assessment of pressure sore development risk;
  - Description of present skin integrity;
  - Description of pressure sore prevention interventions planned and evidence of outcome evaluation;
  - Recommended continued treatment and care.

# Chapter 5: Anatomy and Physiology of the Skin

## Anatomy

The skin is a complex structure. It is the largest organ of the body in terms of surface area. The skin consists of three basic layers of cells:

1.  The *epidermis* is the outer avascular layer of the skin. The cells of the epidermis, the life span of which is approximately 28–30 days, are actually dead and are constantly being shed and replaced by cells from the deeper layers.

2.  The *dermis* is the middle layer of the skin that supports and anchors the epidermis. Complex protein fibres, called collagen fibres, provide strength and elasticity to this layer, which carries blood vessels, nerve endings, hair follicles, sweat glands and lymphatic drainage vessels. The dermis cannot regenerate if destroyed. It heals by the formation of granulation tissue, which is then replaced by scar tissue.

3.  The innermost *subcutaneous*, or fatty, layer carries the larger blood vessels that supply the skin. The thickness of this layer varies considerably, depending on the area of the body it covers and the individual.

There are five main functions of the skin and damage to the skin can interfere with these vital functions:

1.  The skin forms the basic barrier between the body and the environment. This protective function prevents the invasion of harmful bacteria, protects the internal organs from injury, and prevents leakage of vital chemicals and fluids.

2.  There are numerous sensory nerve endings in the skin that warn the body of changing stimuli, such as alterations in

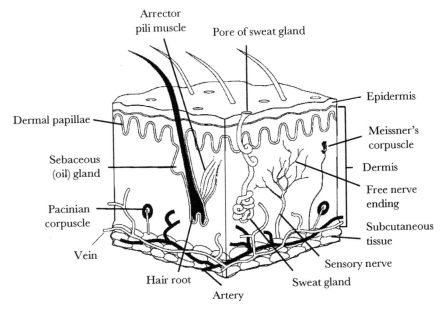

**Figure 5.1** Anatomy of the skin

temperature, touch, pain and pressure. Some end as free nerve endings whilst others have specialised structures, such as Pacinian and Meissner's corpuscles. This function is also linked to the skin's protective role.

3.  The skin has a role in regulating body temperature. It serves to either conserve or distribute body heat according to need, as indicated by the heat regulatory centre in the hypothalamus of the brain. The blood vessels of the skin dilate to increase blood flow, allowing heat to be lost, or constrict to reduce blood flow in order to conserve body heat. Activity of sweat glands also varies with changes in the calibre of the blood vessels.

4.  The subcutaneous layer of the skin acts as a store for water and fat metabolism. This provides insulation and protects the underlying muscle and bone against mechanical forces. It also provides an essential nutritional store.

5.  The skin is not completely airtight and a certain amount of gaseous exchange occurs. The skin absorbs ultraviolet radiation, which aids the conversion of sterol substances to vitamin D.

# Physiology

As with any tissue, a healthy blood supply is essential for its survival. The blood vessels of the skin are perhaps its most vulnerable structures, and certainly the most significant when considering pressure sore formation. The heart pumps oxygen-rich blood from the lungs to all areas of the body, via the arteries. The arteries branch to form small arterioles, which themselves branch into tiny capillaries. The capillaries form a network that brings blood close to each cell in the body, including the skin. The skin receives up to one third of the body's circulating blood. These capillaries are approximately 8 micrometres in diameter and their walls consist of a single layer of very thin cells through which oxygen and other essential nutrients may be passed into the surrounding cells. This structure also allows carbon dioxide and other harmful waste products to filter back into the circulation for excretion. The capillaries rejoin to form venules, which in turn join up to form larger veins that carry deoxygenated blood back to the heart. Average blood pressure in the arteries of a healthy individual at rest is around 120/80 millimetres of mercury (mmHg). The upper figure is the systolic pressure, the high pressure produced when the heart is contracting. The lower figure is the diastolic pressure which is maintained in the arteries between heart beats by elastic recoil of the arterial walls. As blood flows around the body, arterial blood pressure drops. This is because of increased resistance to flow through the much narrower arterioles and capillaries. Landis (1930) undertook important work that examined blood pressure in the capillaries of healthy individuals. He found that the average pressure of blood flow at the arteriolar end of the capillary was 32 mmHg, decreasing to an average of 12 mmHg at the venous end, with a mean capillary pressure of 20 mmHg. Capillary closing pressure represents the degree of pressure required to occlude the capillary and interrupt blood flow. Although not an absolute value, it is thought that external pressures above the average mean capillary blood pressure of 20 mmHg will cause capillary closure, and therefore may precipitate the development of a pressure sore (Bader and Gant, 1988; Landis, 1930; Schubert and Fagrell, 1989). Capillary closing pressure in individuals experiencing ill health can be much lower than 20 mmHg (Landis, 1930), therefore increasing an individual's vulnerability to tissue damage from external pressure.

## Summary points

- The skin is the body's largest organ in terms of surface area
- The skin is a complex structure. It comprises three layers:

- epidermis
  dermis
  subcutaneous tissue
- Damage to the skin will interfere with its vital functions:
  protection
  sensation
  heat regulation
  storage
  absorption
- The skin's blood supply is the most important of its structures when considering the formation of pressure sores
- Capillary closing pressure represents the degree of pressure required to occlude the capillary and interrupt blood flow
- Landis (1930) found that the average mean capillary blood pressure in healthy individuals is 20 mmHg
- Although not an absolute value, it is thought that external pressures above 20 mmHg will cause capillary closure, and therefore may precipitate the development of a pressure sore
- Landis (1930) recognised that capillary closing pressure in individuals experiencing ill health can be much lower than 20 mmHg

# Chapter 6: Aetiology of Pressure Sores

Definition of a Pressure Sore:

'A localised area of cellular damage resulting either from direct pressure on the skin causing ischaemia, or from shearing or friction forces causing mechanical stress on the tissues' (Chapman and Chapman, 1986).

As identified in the above definition of a pressure sore, tissue damage can occur as a result of one or more of the following forces, which have been identified as significant *precipitating* factors in the development of pressure sores:

- pressure
- friction
- shearing

Furthermore, many *predisposing* factors are thought to increase an individual's vulnerability to tissue damage as a result of these precipitating factors. For example, a healthy individual may be exposed to pressure, shear or friction and not sustain tissue damage as a result of this, whilst conversely, a susceptible individual may sustain tissue damage due to a combination of predisposing factors that greatly increase his or her vulnerability to the effects of pressure, shear or friction. Predisposing factors can be classified as those that are intrinsic and extrinsic. Intrinsic factors are those aspects relating to an individual's mental and physical condition that are considered to increase his or her susceptibility to tissue damage, such as nutritional status and cardiovascular function. Extrinsic factors include all external influences on an individual's tissue viability, such as the effect of drugs and other treatment regimens and personal hygiene.

Holistic, accurate and ongoing individual assessment in order to identify the presence of any of these intrinsic and extrinsic predisposing factors is therefore of key importance in the prevention of pressure sores (see chapter 7 Risk Assessment and chapter 8 Preventative Management for details of these predisposing factors).

## Physiology of Tissue Damage from Pressure

Pressure damage occurs when skin and other tissues are directly compressed between bone and another surface. Capillary closing pressure represents the degree of external pressure required to occlude the blood vessels and thus to interrupt blood flow. It is thought that external pressures above the mean capillary blood pressure will cause capillary closure (Bader and Gant, 1988; Landis, 1930; Schubert and Fagrell, 1989). Landis (1930) found that the average mean capillary blood pressure in healthy individuals was 20 mmHg. He also recognised that it can be much lower in individuals experiencing ill health. Interruption of blood flow causes tissue ischaemia, which results in a deficiency of oxygen supply to the cells, known as hypoxia, and a build up of toxic metabolic waste.

External pressure sufficient to interrupt blood flow to the skin causes blanching; a normal process where lack of blood makes the skin appear paler. In normal circumstances, removal of the external pressure gives rise to a temporary erythema, caused by reactive hyperaemia. This is increased blood flow to an area of tissue that was formerly ischaemic, and is characterised by a temporary red flush to the area. Normal skin colour is restored quickly. However, if external pressure is maintained for too long, or if the circulation is otherwise compromised, the local tissue cells will be damaged and begin to die. Erythema will be noted but, instead of being caused by reactive hyperaemia, this skin reddening is caused by blood leaking from the damaged capillaries and normal skin colour will not be restored.

## Characteristics of Pressure and its Relationship to Tissue Damage

The relationship between exposure to pressure and tissue damage is dependent on two characteristics of the pressure:

- intensity of the pressure
- duration of the pressure

The intensity of pressure refers to the degree of pressure, whereas the duration of pressure refers to the length of exposure to that pressure.

Reswick and Rogers (1976) demonstrated that exposure to low pressure can cause tissue damage if it is sustained over several hours, whereas exposure to very high pressure can cause tissue damage within minutes. Other authors (Dinsdale, 1973; Groth, 1942) have also demonstrated this inverse relationship between duration and intensity of pressure in relation to pressure sore formation (Figure 6.1).

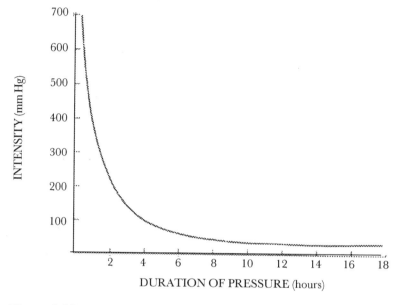

**Figure 6.1** Inverse relationship between duration and intensity of pressure

A study by Kosiak (1959) found that tissues could withstand pressures as high as 400 mmHg without signs of damage, whilst tissues stressed with much less pressure developed irreversible damage. Although 400 mmHg is an extremely high pressure, it was relieved periodically throughout the trial. The lower pressure was held unrelieved against the tissues. The results of this study firmly indicate that tissue damage caused by pressure is largely influenced by the duration of the applied pressure. The effect of pressure has also been found to be cumulative; repeated short periods of occlusion may be as damaging as a single long period of occlusion (Brand, 1976).

## Tissue Interface Pressure

Tissue interface pressure refers to the intensity of pressure to which tissues are exposed by any surface in contact with them. The lower the interface pressure the lower the pressure on the tissue capillaries. As identified earlier in this chapter, external pressure of approximately 20 mmHg can be sufficient to cause capillary occlusion in a healthy individual. Interface pressures are transmitted to the bone through all intermediate tissue. Deep internal pressure can be three to five times greater than surface interface pressure, and can therefore cause extensive deep internal tissue damage with no immediate epidermal damage apparent. This phenomenon is described as the cone of pressure principle. Damage may occur deep in the tissues and may not be visibly apparent for 1–2 weeks after the initial injury (David, 1987). Hence, some sores appear to deteriorate quite dramatically shortly after epidermal damage is first observed. Tissue damage can therefore be prevented by consideration of the intensity and duration of pressure to which a patient is exposed.

The standard hospital foam mattress can produce interface pressures of approximately 130 mmHg (Department of Health, 1993a). The use of such a support system for an individual who is at risk of pressure sore development is therefore clearly inadequate. Interface pressure measurements are subject to inaccuracy because the pressure-measuring device will violate the interface it is intended to measure. In light of this, such measures will only be indicators of interface pressures and, as such, it is recommended that caution is exercised with suggested absolute values.

## Physiology of Tissue Damage from Friction

Skin damage caused by friction typically occurs when the skin has rubbed against another surface, for example, elbows and heels rubbing against a sheet. An individual's exposure to friction is typically the result of poor lifting or handling techniques, either on the part of the individual him or herself or a carer. Friction causes the epidermis to be stripped away, and therefore commonly causes shallow dermal ulcers or blisters. Friction sores are usually painful but relatively superficial, although they can make the skin more vulnerable to pressure damage. Tissue damage resulting from friction forces can therefore be prevented by good lifting and handling techniques.

## Physiology of Tissue Damage from Shear

Shear occurs when tissues are wrenched in opposite directions, resulting in disruption or angulation of capillary blood vessels. Shear occurs most commonly in individuals who spend long periods of

time in a semi-recumbent position, for example,
slowly slips down the bed and the outer layer of t
mis, remains static but the underlying tissues a
Eventually, this relative movement causes stretc
tion of the capillary blood vessels and tissue isch;
can cause full-thickness tissue damage, and is ar
tating factor in the development of many sacral and heel pressure
sores (Bader and Gant, 1988). Tissue damage resulting from shearing forces can therefore be prevented by good positioning.

## Location of Pressure Sores

Pressure sores can occur anywhere on the body, however most occur
over bony prominences where there is less protection afforded by the
tissue layers. The bony prominences affected can be any of those that
support the body during lying, sitting and standing. Among the highest percentage of pressure sores are those occurring on the sacrum
and buttocks (Dealey, 1991; Torrance, 1983). With this in mind,
consideration should be given to seating surfaces in addition to lying
surfaces.

## Classification of Pressure Sores

Pressure sores represent a continuum from an erythematous area of
skin to an open wound extending deep into the tissue. (See chapter
11 for more information on the classification of pressure sores.)

## Summary points

- There are three significant precipitating factors in the development of pressure sores:
     pressure
     shear
     friction
- Furthermore, many intrinsic and extrinsic predisposing
  factors are thought to increase an individual's vulnerability to
  tissue damage as a result of these precipitating factors
- Holistic, accurate and on-going patient assessment in order to
  identify the presence of any of these intrinsic and extrinsic
  predisposing factors is of key importance in the prevention of
  pressure sores

The relationship between exposure to pressure and tissue damage is dependent on two characteristics of the pressure:
- intensity
- duration

- Many authors have demonstrated an inverse relationship between duration and intensity of pressure (Dinsdale, 1973; Groth, 1942; Reswick and Rogers, 1976)
- The effect of pressure has also been found to be cumulative; repeated short periods of occlusion may be as damaging as a single long period of occlusion (Brand, 1976)
- Deep internal pressures can be three to five times greater than surface interface pressures causing deep internal tissue damage with no immediate epidermal damage apparent for 1–2 weeks after the initial injury (David, 1987). This is the cone of pressure principle
- Tissue damage caused by friction occurs when the epidermis rubs against another surface
- Tissue damage from shearing forces occurs when tissues are wrenched in opposite directions, resulting in disruption or angulation of capillary blood vessels
- The majority of pressure sores occur over bony prominences, with the highest percentage occurring on the sacrum and buttocks (Dealey, 1991; Torrance, 1983)
- Pressure sores represent a continuum from an erythematous epidermal area to an open wound extending into deep tissue (See chapter 11 for more information on the classification of pressure sores)

# Chapter 7:
# Risk Assessment

The aim of patient assessment is to identify and explore factors that may predispose a patient to tissue damage from pressure, shear and friction so that comprehensive measures can be introduced to the patient's care and treatment.

The range of predisposing factors that contribute to the development of tissue damage are examined in Chapter 8 Preventative Management. However, it is clear that there is little consensus in relation to the key prognostic factors associated with the development of pressure sores, (Bridel, 1994; Vohra and McCollum, 1994).

## Pressure Sore Risk Assessment Tools

It has been reported that there are some 17 pressure sore risk assessment tools in existence, many of which have not been subjected to thorough evaluation (Clarke and Farrar, 1991, cited in Edwards, 1994). Four of these risk assessment tools have been selected for brief review, the aim of which is to provide the reader with information regarding the tools' inherent strengths and weaknesses.

The principal authors of these tools are:

- Norton (1962)
- Waterlow (1985)
- Braden (1987)
- Lowthian (1976)

The tools have been selected on the basis that they are frequently used and therefore widely documented (Johnson, 1994). The tools are British in origin with the exception of Braden which originates from the USA. Although the Braden tool is less well known in the UK, it is considered to have greater reliability and validity than either the Norton or Waterlow tool (Bridel, 1994). The tool developed by Lowthian at the Royal National Orthopaedic Hospital, Stanmore, is known as the Pressure Sore Prediction Score, PSPS, and is designed for use primarily within an orthopaedic setting.

## Predictors or Indicators?

The predictive ability of a tool, that is its ability to predict those patients who may develop a pressure sore (i.e. sensitivity) and those patients who may not develop a pressure sore (i.e. specificity), is clearly important in circumstances where human and material resources are deployed on the basis of a pressure sore risk assessment score. However, most authors agree that risk assessment tools should not be used as the basis for patient management decisions, and should take second place to the clinical judgement of the nurse and the multidisciplinary team (Norton, 1988, cited in Flanagan, 1993; Waterlow, 1987). Research undertaken to assess the sensitivity and specificity of various risk assessment tools indicates that all tools have some shortcomings in terms of predictive ability. Risk assessment tools may consequently be more accurately described as indicators than predictors.

## Research Base of Risk Assessment Tools

The components of all risk assessment tools have been determined by a review of the literature pertaining to pressure sores, and/or on the basis of clinical experience and judgement (Bridel, 1994). No one risk assessment tool may therefore be said to be truly research based. Bridel (1994) states that there are two fundamental limitations to the risk assessment tools detailed in current literature. These are, firstly, the lack of certainty in relation to the prognostic factors identified within the tool and, secondly, the weighting attached both within and between each of these factors. Scientific, and in some cases mathematical, evaluations of some of the published risk assessment tools have been published (for example, Lowthian, 1993; Shakespeare, 1994). However, the contribution made by such publications is limited as data are discussed solely within the context of patient risk score, and patient outcomes in terms of pressure sore development. Nursing interventions (which, it must be argued, are powerful determinants of patient outcomes) are not considered within these types of evaluations, and hence limit their usefulness.

# The Norton Risk Assessment Tool

### Initial Tool Development

The Norton risk assessment tool was developed as a result of systematic observations of elderly hospital patients by Norton (1962), who sought to establish which of a patient's health characteristics were relevant in terms of the development of pressure sores. The data collected suggested that the important characteristics were general physical condition, mental state, activity, mobility and incontinence, and these factors form the basis of the tool (Figure 7.1).

### Risk Score Threshold

The tool is used to derive an overall risk score related to the patient's potential for the development of a pressure sore. A low score indicates a high risk of developing a pressure sore and, similarly, a high score indicates that a patient's likelihood of developing a pressure sore is low. Initial use of the tool by the Norton research team suggested that a score of 12 or below indicated that the patient was very likely to develop a pressure sore. However, this figure was subsequently revised and a score of 14 was considered to be the risk threshold score (Flanagen, 1993). However Spenceley (1988, cited in Williams, 1992)

## THE NORTON SCORE

| (A) Physical condition | (B) Mental state | (C) Activity | (D) Mobility | (E) Incontinence |
|---|---|---|---|---|
| Good 4 | Alert 4 | Ambulant 4 | Full 4 | None 4 |
| Fair 3 | Apathetic 3 | Walks with help 3 | Slightly limited 3 | Occasional 3 |
| Poor 2 | Confused 2 | Chairbound 2 | Very limited 2 | Usually urinary 2 |
| Very bad 1 | Stuporous 1 | Bedfast 1 | Immobile 1 | Double 1 |

Instructions for use:
1. Assess the patient's condition and score accordingly (1–4) under each heading (A–E)
2. Total the scores together
3. A total of 14 and below indicates a patient is at risk and preventative measures should be taken. The lower the total, the higher the risk
4. Assess the patient regularly

**Figure 7.1** The Norton score. Reproduced by kind permission of Churchill Livingstone

reports that Norton herself has since suggested that a score of 15 or 16 should be used to consider a patient as 'at risk'.

## Strengths and Limitations

The Norton tool has received widespread critical review. It has been shown to over-predict and to under-predict patients who are at risk of developing pressure sores (Flanagan, 1993). Under-prediction was reported to occur when the tool was used for patients who were either undergoing surgery (Lincoln et al., 1986, ibid), or recovering from myocardial infarction (Pritchard, 1986, ibid). A further criticism of the Norton tool is that it is said to be crude, in that it fails to encompass the full range of aetiological factors that are relevant in pressure sore formation (Barratt, cited in Williams, 1992). Similarly, the tool has often been criticised for its failure to include pain and nutrition categories. However, Norton claims that the exclusion of the nutrition category was not an oversight, and that it was assumed that the patient's nutritional status would be reflected in the general condition of the individual (Norton, 1988, cited in Flanagan, 1993). Norton also felt that, at the time when the tool was developed, nurses did not necessarily possess the skills required to undertake nutritional assessments of patients. Finally, an important criticism of the Norton tool is that users have reported difficulty in determining the internal ratings of the tool items. For example, Lincoln (1986) reported that independent nursing assessors experienced difficulty in agreeing on the rating of a given patient's physical condition (good, fair, poor, very bad). However, another study also found that student nurses were slightly better able to agree on the risk score for a given patient when using the Norton scale than they were when using the Waterlow scale (Dealey, 1989, cited in Bridel, 1994).

## Summary

The Norton risk assessment tool is well known and widely used. The first pressure sore risk assessment tool of its kind, it is based on systematic observations of elderly patients who developed pressure sores during their hospital stay. Use of the tool within elderly care settings would therefore appear to be appropriate. The tool's validity and reliability have been repeatedly investigated, although the results of such investigations have in some cases been inconsistent. The problem of assessor subjectivity is apparent in this relatively simple tool. The use of assessment guidelines or operational definitions of the sub-category ratings would enable the effect of rater subjectivity to be minimised.

# The Waterlow Risk Assessment Tool

### Initial Tool Development

It appears that the Waterlow pressure sore risk assessment tool was developed following a review of research that had been conducted on pressure sores and discussions with medical colleagues (Waterlow, 1985, cited in Bridel, 1994). The tool was designed to act as a practical 'aide-memoire' for nurses working within medical and surgical settings. The aim of the tool was twofold. Firstly, it was to provide guidelines on the selection of preventative aids and equipment as well as on the management of established pressure sores. Secondly, it aimed to promote the user's awareness of the causes of pressure sores and provide a means of determining risk of pressure sore development (Waterlow, 1985, cited in Bridel, 1993). In contrast to the other authors of tools described in this section, it appears that Waterlow did not undertake any data collection to support the developmental stage of her work.

### Risk Score Threshold

The scoring system incorporates six main areas of risk:

- build/weight
- continence
- skin type
- mobility
- sex/age
- appetite

In addition, a special risk section alerts the user to tissue malnutrition, neurological deficit, surgery/trauma and specific medication (Figure 7.2).

The risk score threshold is 10, however, above this threshold, there are degrees of risk identified that relate to the score. A score of 10–15 is considered 'at risk', a score of 15–20 as 'high risk', and a score of 20 or above as 'very high risk'. As stated, however, there does not appear to have been any work on the part of the author in terms of establishing the validity of the risk score scheme.

### Strengths and Limitations

The fact that the tool was developed to be used in both medical and surgical settings means that the tool requires a more in-depth patient

## Waterlow Pressure Sore Prevention/Treatment Policy

RING SCORES IN TABLE, ADD TOTAL. SEVERAL SCORES PER CATEGORY CAN BE USED

| Build/Weight for Height | * | Skin Type | * | Sex/Age | * | Special Risks | * |
|---|---|---|---|---|---|---|---|
| Average | 0 | Healthy | 0 | Male | 1 | **Tissue Malnutrition** | * |
| Above Average | 1 | Tissue Paper | 1 | Female | 2 | e.g. Terminal Cachexia | 8 |
| Obese | 2 | Dry |  | 14–49 | 1 | Cardiac Failure | 5 |
| Below Average | 3 | Oedematous |  | 50–64 | 2 | Peripheral Vascular Disease | 5 |
|  |  | Clammy (Temp↑) |  | 65–74 | 3 | Anaemia | 2 |
|  |  | Discoloured | 2 | 75–80 | 4 | Smoking | 1 |
|  |  | Broken/Spot | 3 | 81+ | 5 |  |  |

| Continence | * | Mobility | * | Appetite | * | Neurological Deficit | * |
|---|---|---|---|---|---|---|---|
| Complete/Catheterised | 0 | Fully | 0 | Average | 0 | e.g. Diabetes, M.S., CVA, Motor/Sensory Paraplegia | 4–6 |
| Occasionally Incontinent | 1 | Restless/Fidgety | 1 | Poor | 1 |  |  |
| Cath/Incontinent of Faeces | 2 | Apathetic | 2 | N.G. Tube/Fluids only | 2 | **Major Surgery/Trauma** | * |
| Doubly Incontinent | 3 | Restricted | 3 | NBM/Anorexic | 3 | Orthopaedic Below Waist, Spinal | 5 |
|  |  | Inert/Traction | 4 |  |  | on Table 2 hours | 5 |
|  |  | Chairbound | 5 |  |  |  |  |
|  |  |  |  |  |  | **Medication** | * |
|  |  |  |  |  |  | Cytotoxics High Dose steroids Anti-Inflammatory | 4 |

| Score | 10+ A Risk | 15+ High Risk | 20+ Very High Risk |
|---|---|---|---|

Remember tissue damage often starts prior to admission, in casualty. A seated patient is also at risk.

Assessment: If the patient falls into any of the risk categories then preventative nursing techniques and preventative aids will definitely be necessary.

PREVENTATIVE AIDS:

Special Mattress/Bed: 10+ overlays or specialist foam mattresses.
15+ alternating pressure overlays, mattresses and bed systems.
20+ Bed System: Fluidised, bead, low air loss and alternating pressure mattresses.
Note: Preventative aids cover a wide spectrum of specialist features. Efficacy should be judged, if possible, on the basis of independent evidence.

Cushions: No patient should sit in a wheelchair without some form of cushioning. If nothing else is available — use the patient's own pillow.
10+4" Foam cushion.
15+ Specialist cell and/or foam cushion
20+ Cushion capable of adjustment to suit individual patient.

Bed Clothing: Avoid plastic draw sheets, inco pads and tightly tucked in sheets/sheet covers, especially when using Specialist bed and mattress overlay systems.
Use Duvet-plus vapour permeable cover.

## NURSING CARE

General: Frequent changes of position, lying/sitting
Use of pillows

Pain Appropriate pain control
Nutrition High protein, vitamins, minerals
Patient Handling: Correct lifting technique – Hoists – Monkey Pole – Transfer Devices
Patient Comfort Aids: Real sheepskins — Bed Cradle
Operating Table
Theatre/A&E Trolley 4" cover plus adequate protection.
Skin Care: General Hygiene, NO rubbing, cover with an appropriate dressing

**If treatment is required, first remove pressure**

## WOUND CLASSIFICATION

Stirling Pressure Score severity scale (SPSSS)

**Stage 0** — No clinical evidence of pressure sore
**0.1** — Healed with scarring
**0.2** — Tissue damage not assessed as a pressure sore (a) below

**Stage 1** — Discoloration of intact skin
**1.1** — Non-blanchable erythema with increased local heat
**1.2** — Blue/purple/black discoloration — the sore is at least **Stage 1** (a or b)

**Stage 2** — Partial thickness skin loss or damage
**2.1** — Blister
**2.2** — Abrasion
**2.3** — Shallow ulcer, no undermining of adjacent tissue
**2.4** — Any of these with underlying blue/purple/black discoloration or induration. The sore is at least **Stage 2** (a, b or c+d for **2.3**, +e for **2.4**)

**Stage 3** — Full-thickness skin loss involving damage/necrosis of subcutaneous tissue, not extending to underlying bone tendon or joint capsule
**3.1** — Crater, without undermining adjacent tissue
**3.2** — Crater, with undermining of adjacent tissue
**3.3** — Sinus, the full extent of which is uncertain
**3.4** — Necrotic tissue masking full extent of damage.
The sore is at least **Stage 3** (b, +/-e, f, g, +h for **3.4**)

**Stage 4** — Full-thickness loss with extensive destruction and tissue necrosis extending to underlying bone tendon or capsule
**4.1** — Visible exposure of bone tendon or capsule
**4.2** — Sinus assessed as extending to same (b+/-e, f, g, h, i)

Guide to types of Dressings/Treatment
a. Semipermeable membrane
b. Hydrocolloid
c. Foam dressing
d. Alginate
e. Hydrogel
f. Alginate rope/ribbon
g. Foam cavity filler
h. Enzymatic debridement
i. Surgical debridement

**Figure 7.2** The Waterlow Pressure Sore Prevention/Treatment Policy. Reproduced with kind permission of Mrs Judy Waterlow

assessment, as it encompasses a broad range of important risk factors, such as nutritional status and tissue tolerance, which some other scales, for example Norton, do not include. The tool is also said to have been designed to provide flexibility for nurses who feel that they would like to make the tool more specific to their needs by adding sub-categories with associated scores to the tool (Flanagen, 1993). Modification of the Waterlow tool has been undertaken by several users, for example, Johnson (1994) describes the changes made to the tool prior to its use in a neurological setting. An additional advantage conferred by the tool is that the differentiation between different levels of patient risk status allows the user to gauge the previously vague concept of risk status and plan preventative measures which are appropriate for such a level of risk (Flanagan, 1993). Gross over-prediction of patients at risk using this tool has been reported by various authors (for example, Dealey, 1989, cited in Bridel, 1993), and reliability of the tool has also been shown to be poor, comparing unfavourably to that of the Norton tool in this respect.

## Summary

The tool has enjoyed widespread popularity due to the fact that it is accompanied by preventative and treatment guidelines for pressure sores, and so offers an educational component. Consequently, it has been incorporated into many healthcare providers' pressure sore prevention strategies. However, the fact that little has been achieved in the way of formal evaluation of this tool reduces its scientific credibility.

As identified with the Norton tool, the apparently poor inter-rater reliability of the tool could be improved if operational definitions or more detailed assessment guidelines were made available to users.

# The Braden Risk Assessment Tool

## Initial Tool Development

Braden and Bergstrom's risk assessment tool (1987) is said to have been based on a conceptualisation of the aetiological factors relating to pressure sore formation (Braden and Bergstrom, 1989, cited in Bridel, 1994). The tool is composed of six categories: sensory perception, moisture, activity, mobility, nutrition, and friction and shear (Figure 7.3). Publications by the authors indicate that evaluations of the efficacy of this tool have taken place in both surgical, medical and intensive therapy units (Bergstrom, 1976, cited in Salvadelena et al., 1992).

**Risk Score Threshold**

The range of scores obtained from this tool is from 6 to 23. A score of 16 or below is said to indicate that a patient is at risk of developing a pressure sore. There are no identified levels of risk within the scale.

**Strengths and Limitations**

Because the internal ratings of the six categories are supported by assessment guidelines, which seek to clearly describe the behaviour and/or experiences of the patient, the inter-rater reliability of the tool should, in theory, be superior to both the Norton and Waterlow scales, although no comparative work has yet been undertaken. The view that this tool confers good reliability is supported by Bridel (1993), who considers this tool to be the most reliable of those described in the literature. Bergstrom and Braden (1989) reported that in a study of 22 graduate students and registered nurses in a rehabilitation setting in the USA, absolute agreement between scores for given patients was 88%, and +/- one point agreement was found to be 100% (cited in Bridel, 1993). However, Bergstrom and Braden also reported that when licensed practical nurses' and nursing assistants' scores were considered, this reduced the inter-rater reliability. This led the author to recommend that the tool should be used only by registered nurses.

The view expressed by Flanagan (1993) that this tool has demonstrated greater sensitivity and specificity than any other published scale is supported by most of the publications that refer to this tool. An exception to this is a publication by Salvadalena et al. (1992), which fails to identify a statistical correlation between the Braden scale score and pressure sore formation. The fact that the tool requires a detailed patient assessment has been cited as a criticism (Taylor, 1988, cited in Flanagan, 1993) on the basis that it cannot easily be used in the initial period of admission to a given care setting.

**Summary**

The Braden scale has been widely utilised in the USA and this is reflected in the fact that the Agency for Health Care Policy and Research recently recommended it for use in predicting pressure sore development, (Vohra and McCollum, 1994). Evaluations of the tool's reliability and validity have been predominantly favourable. However, the tool is not well known in the UK and practitioners wishing to use it would need to ensure they had a good working knowledge of it prior to implementation.

Patient Name ............... Evaluator's Name ............... Date of Assessment ...............

| | 1 | 2 | 3 | 4 |
|---|---|---|---|---|
| **Sensory Perception** ability to respond meaningfully to pressure-related discomfort | **Completely Limited** Unresponsive (does not moan, flinch or grasp to painful stimuli) due to diminished level of consciousness or sedation OR Limited ability to feel pain over most of body surface | **Very Limited** Responds only to painful stimuli, cannot communicate discomfort except by moaning or restlessness OR Has a sensory impairment which limits the ability to feel pain or discomfort over 1/2 of body | **Slightly Limited** Responds to verbal commands but cannot always communicate discomfort or need to be turned OR Has some sensory impairment which limits ability to feel pain or discomfort in 1 or 2 extremities | **No Impairment** Responds to verbal commands. Has no sensory deficit which would affect ability to feel or voice pain or discomfort |
| **Moisture** degree to which skin is exposed to moisture | **Constantly Moist** Skin is kept moist almost constantly by perspiration, urine, etc. Dampness is detected every time patient is moved or turned | **Very Moist** Skin is often, but not always moist. Linen must be changed at least once a shift | **Occasionally Moist** Skin is occasionally moist, requiring an extra linen change approximately once a day | **Rarely Moist** Skin is usually dry. Linen only requires changing at routine intervals |
| **Activity** degree of physical activity | **Bedfast** Confined to bed | **Chairfast** Ability to walk severely limited or non-existent. Cannot bear own weight and/or must be assisted into chair or wheelchair | **Walks Occasionally** Walks occasionally during day, but for very short distances, with or without assistance. Spends majority of each shift in bed or chair | **Walks Frequently** Walks outside the room at least twice a day and inside room at least once every 2 hours during waking hours |

| | 1 | 2 | 3 | 4 |
|---|---|---|---|---|
| **Mobility** ability to change and control body position | **1. Completely Immobile** Does not make even slight changes in body or extremity position without assistance | **2. Very Limited** Makes occasional slight changes in body or extremity position but unable to make frequent or significant changes independently | **3. Slightly Limited** Makes frequent though slight changes in body or extremity position independently | **4. No Limitation** Makes major and frequent changes in position without assistance |
| **Nutrition** usual food intake pattern | **1. Very Poor** Never eats a complete meal. Rarely eats more than 1/3 of any food offered. Eats 2 servings or less of protein (meat or dairy products) per day. Takes fluids poorly. Does not take a liquid dietary supplement OR Is NBM and/or maintained on clear liquids or IVs for more than 5 days | **2. Probably Inadequate** Rarely eats a complete meal and generally eats only about 1/2 of any food offered. Protein intake includes only 3 servings of meat or dairy products per day. Occasionally will take a dietary supplement OR Receives less than optimum amount of liquid diet or tube feeding | **3. Adequate** Eats over half of most meals. Eats a total of 4 servings of protein (meat, dairy products) each day. Occasionally will refuse a meal, but will usually take a supplement if offered OR Is on a tube feeding or TPN regimen which probably meets most of nutritional needs | **4. Excellent** Eats most of every meal. Never refuses a meal. Usually eats a total of 4 or more servings of meat and dairy products. Occasionally eats between meals. Does not require supplementation |
| **Friction and Shear** | **1. Problem** Requires moderate to maximum assistance in moving. Complete lifting without sliding against sheets is impossible. Frequently slides down in bed or chair, requiring frequent repositioning with maximum assistance. Spasticity, contractures or agitation lead to almost constant friction | **2. Potential Problem** Moves freely or requires minimum assistance. During a move skin probably slides to some extent against sheets. Chair restraints or other devices. Maintains relatively good position in chair or bed most of the time but occasionally slides down | **3. No Apparent Problem** Moves in bed and in chair independently and has sufficient muscle strength to lift up completely during move. Maintains good position in bed or chair at all times | |

**Figure 7.3** Braden scale for predicting pressure sore risk (Bergstrom and Braden, 1987). Reprinted by kind permission of Sage Publications, Inc.

# Pressure Sore Prevention Score (PSPS)

### Initial Tool Development

The PSPS tool was conceived by Lowthian (1976), at the Royal National Orthopaedic Hospital, who has since sought to evaluate its efficacy within the orthopaedic setting.

### Risk Score Threshold

The scheme of the tool is that the nurse/rater is asked a series of questions in relation to the patient's health status. The questions consider six aspects of the patient's condition, asking if he/she is;

- sitting up?
- unconscious?
- of poor general condition?
- incontinent?
- able to lift him/herself up?
- able to walk?

A score of six or above is considered to indicate that the patient is at risk.

### Strengths and Limitations

Lowthian reports that he spent three years collecting data to assess the sensitivity and specificity of the tool (Lowthian 1994, letter to the Editor, Journal of Tissue Viability), and claims these to be good (89% sensitivity, 76% specificity). Whilst the use of the tool in an orthopaedic setting is supported by the author's work, no other evaluations in other settings have been undertaken. Category examples which reflect the response to the questions posed within the tool have been formulated so as to enhance the tool's reliability.

### Summary

The PSPS tool is clearly one which should be considered for use within an orthopaedic setting. Further work would need to be undertaken to establish the tool's suitability for other settings.

## PRESSURE SORE PREVENTION AID

**PSPS** Pressure Sore Prediction Score

| | | NO | No but.. | Yes but.. | YES |
|---|---|---|---|---|---|
| | **S**itting up? (long time) | (0 | 1 | 2 | 3) |
| **"A"** | **U**nconscious? | (0 | 1 | 2 | 3) |
| | **P**oor general condition? | (0 | 1 | 2 | 3) |
| | **I**ncontinent? | (0 | 1 | 2 | 3) |

| | | YES | Yes & No | No | Tick Scores |
|---|---|---|---|---|---|
| | **L**ifts up? | (0 | 1 | 2) | with felt pen |
| **"B"** | **G**ets up & walks? | (0 | 1 | 2) | |
| | | | | | TOTAL |

**"A" & "B"** — Questions on state of patient now:- see notes below

### USUALLY, A TOTAL OF 6 OR MORE MEANS DANGER

### NOTES ON THE PSPS

a)   In part "A"       a "YES" answer gives the greatest risk (3) while "Yes but" gives less risk (2) and "No but" gives a slight risk (1)

b)   In part "B"        a "NO" answer gives the greatest risk (2) while "Yes & No" gives somewhat less risk (1)

**S**itting up? (long time)   Propped up in bed for long periods means a definite "Yes" answer. Sitting in a chair can be risky, but wheelchairs are not as bad as ordinary chairs — for sitting long. On admission decide nursing position to be used

**U**nconscious?   Mental confusion may qualify as a "No but" answer

**P**oor general?   This may be severe/sudden illness or a long standing disability (e.g. paralysis). A lack of response to pain suggests a poor condition, as also does great age

**I**ncontinent?   The main point is how often the patient is wet underneath: although poor bladder/bowel control may also mean that the skin is not healthy. On admission discover if patient was incontinent in last two days

**L**ifts up?   When possible the patient is asked to try, without help from anyone else to "Lift up". A "Yes" answer means that the patient does lift his pelvis clear of the bed (or seat) at the time of asking

**G**ets up & walks?   A "Yes" answer implies normal, or nearly normal walking

**N.B.** Unusual circumstances (in your nursing situation) may call for a slight change in the PSPS danger level (e.g. if many sores are starting and are unexpected reduce the danger level to 5)

Pressure sores are not bound to happen — even if the PSPS is very high

**Figure 7.4** The PSPS. Reproduced with kind permission of Peter Lowthian

| | Answer |
|---|---|
| **Sitting up (Long time)**<br>a)  Bedfast & nursed flat.<br>b)  Only sits up in a chair — short periods.<br>c)  Does not sit for long periods (Ambulant). | **No** |
| a)  Sits in self-propelled chair (less than 10 hours) but flat when in bed. | **No, but..** |
| a)  Sits in self-propelled chair for 10 hours or more.<br>b)  Sits for short periods — both in bed and in fixed chair. | **Yes, but..** |
| a)  Propped up in bed — longish periods — most of the day.<br>b)  Sits up both day and night. | **Yes** |
| **Unconscious**<br>a)  Fully conscious & orientated.<br>b)  Fully conscious & slightly confused. | **No** |
| a)  Confused.<br>b)  Withdrawn.<br>c)  Semiconscious at times. | **No, but..** |
| a)  Rousable — responds to commands or pain | **Yes, but..** |
| a)  Deeply unconscious.<br>b)  Does not respond to pain. | **Yes** |
| **Poor General Condition**<br>a)  Fairly good general condition.<br>b)  Awaiting minor op.<br>c)  Minor problem (mental or physical). | **No** |
| a)  Recent operation (under G.A.).<br>b)  Some restriction of lower extremities.<br>c)  Minor sensory neuropathy.<br>d)  Periph arterial disease.<br>e)  Diabetic.<br>f)  Arthritic.<br>g)  Anorexic.<br>h)  Pyrexial.<br>i)  Hypotensive.<br>j)  On steroids.<br>k)  Chemotherapy.<br>l)  Radiotherapy.<br>m)  Elderly & thin, or obese. | **No, but..** |
| a)  Some injuries to lower half of body, but fair general condition.<br>b)  Severe injuries (lower half) but no restriction of movement.<br>c)  Well established chronic disease/disability.<br>d)  Young paraplegic.<br>e)  Active hemiplegic.<br>f)  Elderly & on steroids. | **Yes, but..** |
| a)  Limited mobility & great age.<br>b)  Severe injuries — including legs/pelvis.<br>c)  Seriously/critically ill.<br>d)  Terminal (acute) illness. | |

| | |
|---|---|
| e) Emaciated/cachetic.<br>f) Severe gen. infection.<br>g) Severe uraemia.<br>h) Multiple pathology.<br>i) Iliac thrombosis.<br>j) Severe M.S.<br>k) Hansen's disease.<br>l) Extensive loss of pain.<br>m) Recent paraplegic.<br>n) Quadraplegic.<br>o) On narcotics (for pain).<br>p) Combined chemotherapy, radiotherapy &/or steroids. | **Yes** |
| **Incontinent**<br>a) No incontinence, & no "Accidents" recently.<br>b) Indwelling cath./stoma, but no leaks/accidents. | **No** |
| a) Sometimes wets bed/spills urinal.<br>b) Occasional accidents with attached urinal.<br>c) Occasional leaks from indwelling catheter.<br>d) Occasional faecal incont. | **No, but..** |
| a) Small amounts & infrequent.<br>b) Urine only & infrequent.<br>c) Faecal (infrequent) but some leaks (cath./urinal). | **Yes, but..** |
| a) Continual dribble/leak.<br>b) Frequent urine/faecal incontinence.<br>c) Doubly incontinent. | **Yes** |
| **Lifts up**<br>a) Lifts all of body clear of support.<br>b) Easily lifts pelvis clear. | **Yes** |
| a) Can only lift pelvis with some effort & soon tires.<br>b) Seldom lifts self.<br>c) Can lift with help.<br>d) Lifts slightly — shuffles along support. | **Yes & no** |
| a) Unable to lift pelvis.<br>b) Can neither help with lift, nor shuffle. | **No** |
| **Gets up & walks**<br>a) Fully ambulant.<br>b) Slight impediment.<br>c) Uses aids with no difficulty. | **Yes** |
| a) Has difficulty walking with aid.<br>b) Walks with help & encouragement.<br>c) Soon tires.<br>d) Can only walk to toilet. | **Yes & No** |
| a) Bedfast.<br>b) Chairfast.<br>c) Stands & shuffles — with help & encouragement. | **No** |

This pressure sore prevention aid was developed at the Royal National Orthopaedic Hospital (NHS) Trust, Stanmore, Middx

**Figure 7.5** PSPS Category examples. Reproduced with kind permission of Peter Lowthian

## Optimising the Risk Assessment Tool

In order to optimise the risk assessment tool which has been selected for use the following recommendations are offered:

Select a tool which is appropriate to the patient group, e.g. care of the elderly, orthopaedic care, etc.

Ensure familiarity with the tool is maintained by all members of the nursing team. This may be achieved by the appropriate display of educational material, and ensuring that all staff who are new to the clinical area are appropriately supported in the use of the tool.

Ensure that risk assessment is undertaken at appropriate times during the patient's hospital stay, especially when a major change in health status has occurred. This may be especially important in elderly patients as Bliss (1990) reports that healthy old people, including those with mobility problems, do not normally develop pressure sores, but that those same patients may become acutely vulnerable following the onset of an intercurrent illness or trauma (cited in Edwards, 1994).

Regularly review the cut-off point used to describe risk threshold by reviewing pressure sore incidence data in conjunction with published literature on the application of the tool. In-house development of a risk assessment tool has been suggested by some authors to be a valuable method of enhancing the usefulness of the tool (Clarke and Farrar, 1991, cited in Edwards, 1994; Department of Health, 1993b).

## Summary points

*   The aim of patient assessment is to identify the presence of predisposing and precipitating factors which may influence the development of pressure sores
*   Pressure sore risk assessment tools provide a method of generating a patient risk score which can then be used to inform decisions made in relation to preventative management
*   The usefulness of the risk assessment tool is directly related to how it is used within a given clinical area

- Users should be aware of the strengths and weaknesses of the risk assessment tool they are using
- Strategies for optimising the usefulness of the tool are as follows:
    Appropriate tool selection
    The use of educational material
    Regular reassessment of the patient
    Review inter-rater reliability
    Review risk threshold scores

# Chapter 8:
# Preventative
# Management

Effective pressure sore prevention is based upon a sound knowledge of the aetiology of pressure sores, combined with holistic observation of the patient and assessment of the impact of their condition on their susceptibility to developing pressure sores. Effective preventative management necessitates the involvement of all of the health care team in identifying risk factors. It only takes the failure of one link in the chain of prevention for a pressure sore to develop.

Tissue damage can occur as a result of one or more precipitating factors — *pressure, shear* or *friction.* Furthermore, many predisposing factors are thought to increase an individual's vulnerability to tissue damage as a result of these precipitating factors. Much research has been done to investigate the factors which predispose an individual to tissue damage. The aetiology of pressure sores is widely accepted as being very complex and multifactorial. Some risk factors are difficult to quantify because it would be unethical to perform studies where the desired outcome was destruction of living human tissue. The prevention of pressure sores will not be achieved unless careful consideration is given to controlling or alleviating factors which predispose an individual to tissue breakdown. In this chapter each of the precipitating and main predisposing factors are considered in depth and strategies suggested to either control or alleviate these factors.

## Mobility

The effect of reduced mobility is considered to be the single most important factor in the development of pressure sores and has been widely researched. Many authors confirm that patients confined to bed or sitting are at significantly greater risk of developing pressure sores because of the effects of pressure and shearing. Berlowitz (1989) describes a fourfold increase in risk of pressure sores in these patients.

The body's own defence against pressure damage is to shift weight frequently whether asleep or awake as a response to sensory stimulation. Any factor which interferes with the sensation of pain or which limits the ability to respond by movement therefore increases the risk of pressure sore development. Exton-Smith (1961) studied overnight movement in a group of 50 elderly patients and related the number of spontaneous movements observed to the subsequent development of pressure sores. He clearly demonstrated that a reduced frequency of spontaneous movement results in a higher incidence of pressure sores, and claimed that less than 20 movements per night should be considered a predisposing factor. Analgesia, sedation, reduced consciousness and nerve damage can reduce an individual's sensation to painful stimuli. Inhibited movement may be due to restriction upon movement, for example from traction, drips and drains, the presence of pain, altered consciousness, reduced motor power, sedation or mental illness. Apathy may also reduce a patient's desire to shift their position regularly.

Tissue interface pressure is the external pressure to which tissues are exposed by any surface which is in contact with them. The lower the interface pressure, the lower the pressure on the tissue capillaries. The relationship between exposure to pressure and tissue damage is dependent on two characteristics of the pressure, *intensity* and *duration* (Groth, 1942; Dinsdale, 1973). Tissue capillary occlusion occurs when tissue interface pressure exceeds the mean capillary blood pressure. This causes tissue ischaemia, which results in tissue hypoxia and a build up of toxic metabolic waste. If this situation is sustained the cells will begin to die. The surface in contact with a person is therefore of paramount importance. The aim of pressure-reducing equipment is to either redistribute pressure equally in order to eliminate high point pressures, to alternate the points of pressure or to provide a constant low pressure. Patients should be taught how to relieve pressure from vulnerable areas when they are in bed or sitting in a chair. Written information should be provided to consolidate verbal advice and education. Patients may require moving aids such as a 'monkey pole' or a pull-up rope. Long periods spent lying on trolleys in the Accident & Emergency department, X-Ray department and in the Operating Theatre are associated with increased risk. Patients at risk should be transferred out of these departments at the earliest opportunity, wherever possible to a pressure-reducing bed.

# Lifting and Handling

Tissue damage from friction typically occurs when the skin has rubbed against another surface, for example, elbows or heels rubbing against a sheet. Friction damage is often a result of poor lifting and handling techniques, used by the individual themselves or a carer. Appropriate lifting and handling techniques should always be used, and the method will depend upon the level of communication between the patient and the lifters and on the patient's physical condition. The patient's level of mobility and appropriate handling techniques to be used should be clearly documented in the patient's plan of care. Further guidance on lifting and handling should be sought from a lifting and handling trainer.

# Positioning

Several authors have emphasised the problem of shearing as a result of inappropriate positioning. Shearing occurs when tissues are wrenched in opposite directions resulting in disruption or angulation of capillary blood vessels. These shearing forces can be very destructive to deep tissues (Bader and Gant, 1988). Shearing occurs most commonly in individuals who spend long periods of time in a semi-recumbent position. The patient may slowly slip down the bed and, whilst the outer layer of skin remains static, the underlying tissues are pushed forward. Eventually this relative movement causes stretching and deformation of the capillary blood vessels and tissue ischaemia occurs. Lateral positions endanger the trochanters which are not normally weight-bearing areas. For patients with existing sores the number of positions available to them may be reduced, depending on the number of intact areas upon which they may lie.

# Frequency of Position Changes

Regular turning has been shown to reduce the incidence of pressure sores by many authors, and its effectiveness can easily be understood in relation to the aetiology of pressure sores. It is very difficult to establish the duration of exposure to pressure which will cause a pressure sore. Many authors have drawn on accepted clinical practice, most commonly quoting 2 hours (for example, Anthony, 1987; Hill, 1992), but this figure seems to be rather arbitrary. Duration of exposure to pressure has been found to have an inverse relationship to the intensity of pressure (Groth, 1942; Dinsdale, 1973). The optimum frequency of position changes will also vary according to the patient's general condition both mentally and physically, the type of bed or chair used and other care and treatment considerations.

### The Skin Tolerance Test

This provides an indication of the amount of time tissue can tolerate sustained pressure without damage. After turning the patient, lightly press with a finger the area of skin upon which the patient has been lying or sitting. Initially the skin should blanch (go white), and then return to its normal colour. The return to normal colour should take no longer than twice the length of time finger pressure was applied. The time taken for this 'reactive hyperaemia' to occur correlates with the previous length of vascular occlusion; this has been shown to be true for occlusion periods up to five minutes (Michel, 1990). If the blanching does not occur, or return of normal colour is delayed, this suggests that capillary damage has occurred, and the frequency of position changes should therefore be increased. It is suggested that where a patient has been identified as at risk of developing pressure sores, the skin tolerance test should be performed 30 minutes after initial positioning and the length of time spent by the patient in one position adjusted according to the findings.

### Turning Charts

Lowthian (1979) described the usefulness of a planned regimen of turning in preventing pressure sores. Berecek (1975) suggested that turning regimens must be rigorously implemented to be effective. A planned regimen for turning and repositioning can be supported by the use of a 24 hour turning chart. Where appropriate, the regimen should be planned with the patient in order to take account of their routine, appointments, rest and sleep preferences, meal times and visitors.

### Positioning in Bed

Natural body alignment and patient comfort must be maintained at each position change. The 30 degree tilt position, for example, distributes weight through the soft gluteal muscles which can tolerate pressure up to 3 times longer than tissue over bony prominences (Preston, 1988). To test how effective a new position is at relieving pressure, a hand or arm can be inserted between the patient and the supporting surface. This provides an indication as to how much pressure is being exerted on the patient whilst in a given position. Further advice on positioning may be sought from a physiotherapist.

### Positioning in a Seat

To ensure that a patient is sitting correctly, the following should be observed:

- the patient's bottom should be as far back in the seat as possible
- where possible, the thigh should be supported along its full length
- the hips, knees and ankles should be approximately at 90 degrees (right angles)
- the lumbar spine should be supported
- where a leg rest is used the total height of the leg rest (including pillow if used) should be level with the seat
- the heel should be clear of the leg rest
- where a patient has difficulty in maintaining a position, pillows may be used to provide extra support

Further advice may be sought from an occupational therapist or physiotherapist.

## Nutrition

Much has been written on the role of nutrition in the aetiology of pressure sores.

Certain body characteristics can affect the distribution of pressure over the body's surface. Thin people with little subcutaneous fat and poor muscle bulk often have little padding over bony prominences, which serve as foci for high pressure points. The general scarcity of fat and muscle bulk to dissipate pressure means that pressure is more intense in any one area (Torrance, 1983). At the other extreme, obese people have more fatty padding which gives a more even distribution of pressure; however fatty tissue is poorly vascularised, less resilient and more subject to shearing forces (Torrance, 1983).

Protein is widely reported to be an important dietary element in relation to pressure sore development (for example, Moolten, 1972; Breslow, 1993). The elderly have been shown to have a greater protein requirement (Tuttle, 1965). Vitamin deficiency leads to a reduced integrity of cell walls, decreased enzyme activity for cellular development, and reduced tissue restoration. Vitamin C deficiency has been identified as a factor in pressure sore development. Goode et al. (1992) and Cohen (1968) suggested that zinc deficiency is also an important factor. Anaemia, which may result from a dietary deficiency in either iron or vitamin B12, results in poor blood oxygenation which predisposes tissue death when exposed to pressure (Livesley, 1990). Poor hydration through low fluid intake or high fluid loss from excessive diuretic therapy, diarrhoea, vomiting, blood loss, uncontrolled diabetes, burns etc. reduces tissue resistance and elasticity and thus tissue viability (Livesley, 1990).

Numerous studies have shown that many hospital patients are malnourished (for example, Larsson et al., 1990; Lennard-Jones, 1992). The patients in hospital affected by malnutrition are not a unified group. Patients range from the very young to the very old. They comprise temporary or permanent sufferers of ill health involving any body system. Malnutrition may occur because an individual will not, or cannot, eat or because food is poorly absorbed. It may also occur because of physical disability, such as arthritis, motor neurone disease or multiple sclerosis, where the individual is unable to prepare or eat meals. Malnutrition may arise from an individual's social circumstances, such as poverty or a chaotic home which may limit meals. It may also occur as a result of lack of education about an appropriate diet. Food may be unpalatable for an individual with loss of taste or poor appetite, alternatively it may be unsuitable for an individual with a painful mouth or who has difficulty in chewing. An 'average' appetite is considered to equate to the consumption of three balanced meals per day. Chronic pain, depression or apathy can all lead to loss of interest in food. In hospital food intake may be insufficient because meals are missed due to multiple procedures requiring temporary starvation, or because meals are served in a way which takes no account of a physical disability or feeding difficulty.

Surgical procedures in which a major proportion of the small intestine is removed and disorders of the intestinal muscle or mucosa may give rise to reduced absorption of food, leading to malnutrition.

Nutritional assessment is of paramount importance in order to identify appropriate means of nutritional support which can result in a reduced risk of developing pressure sores. An individual's nutritional requirements will depend on many factors, such as age, gender, weight, body type, activity and stress levels. An individual may need assistance with eating and drinking, a special diet, provision of nutrition via an alternative route, education or any number of other interventions. Meals must be nutritious, but attractively presented to stimulate the appetite. This may involve catering to individual preferences. A dietician can help to plan a suitable diet. It is important that a nutritional assessment of all patients is made as part of their initial medical and nursing assessment. The nutritional status of all patients should be reassessed weekly thereafter.

## Hygiene and Clothing

Inability to maintain safe standards of hygiene may be due to disability, mental status or even socioeconomic problems. Skin exposed to excessive moisture is known to increase the risk of tissue damage. Maceration is the term given to the condition of skin which has become oversaturated with moisture. Maceration causes the skin to become thin, which in turn increases the likelihood of skin abrasion or excoriation. Incontinence is commonly cited as an important risk factor but research findings are inconclusive as to the relative significance regarding pressure sore development. However, moisture and acid from urine and faeces can cause skin maceration and tissue damage from friction becomes more likely (Kelly, 1994).

Norton (1962) found that 39% of incontinent patients developed pressure sores, as opposed to 7% of continent patients. Control of incontinence is important for patient comfort and morale, as well as its contribution in the prevention of maceration. Overuse of pads, plastic sheets and drawsheets to protect the bed can undermine any pressure-reducing properties. A support system designed to be resistant to urine contamination and which is easily cleaned is preferable to one that needs protection with pads and sheets. Overflow incontinence from faecal impaction can also be a problem, and it is possible that a hard faecal bulk in the rectum may affect pressure distribution (Torrance, 1983). The problem can be relieved by use of regular aperients and additional dietary fibre, as well as by suppositories, enemata and manual evacuation. Pressure-relieving cushions for the toilet seat are available from some equipment suppliers.

The skin has a barrier of epidermal lipids, sebum and sweat from the skin glands. This barrier is relatively impermeable to water, however excessive washing, and particularly the use of soap, can strip away this protection. The removal of this barrier encourages skin dehydration and increases the frictional coefficient. Skin has an acid pH which, when washed with soap, can shift to alkaline, causing skin dryness. Skin should therefore be washed as little as possible. It should be kept socially clean, but over-washing avoided. Where cleansing of the skin is necessary, a mild soap or a neutral cleanser should be used. Skin should be dried thoroughly after washing using a patting motion, particularly over vulnerable areas. A rubbing motion should be avoided as this has been associated with deep tissue damage. Dyson (1978) examined the effects of rubbing vulnerable areas of skin. He reported a 38% reduction in the incidence of pressure sores in a control group of patients whose skin was not rubbed compared with that in a group of patients whose skin was rubbed. The practice of rubbing a reddened area to stimulate circulation is considered dubious. Blanching erythema is a sign of reactive hyperaemia, which is an increased flow of blood to an area released from compression. Non-blanching erythema is indicative of damage to the microcirculation and rubbing will only increase the mechanical trauma to the damaged tissue.

Numerous lotions, creams and sprays are advocated for pressure sore prevention. However, few have been clinically evaluated. The use of astringents, such as methylated spirits and alcohol, and witch hazel are potentially harmful as they dry the skin by removing the protective barrier, and can cause vasoconstriction which increases susceptibility to pressure sores in already ischaemic areas (Norton, 1962). The use of barrier creams may help to give protection from the patient's own excreta. Baird (1979) found that when large stock pots of cream were used contamination with *Pseudomonas aerginosa* and *Staphylococcus aureus* was as high as 93%. Contamination of small individual pots or tubes was found to be only 9%. Talcum powder should not be used on vulnerable areas because of its tendency to cake, thereby increasing the likelihood of friction. Powder on the skin also inhibits the ability of the skin to excrete waste products.

Skin should be kept well hydrated as skin that is flaky, cracked or appears dehydrated is more susceptible to damage. Dehydration should be corrected with an increased fluid intake and a moisturising agent, such as aqueous cream, which can also be used as a cleanser instead of soap in bath or wash water or applied topically to dry skin.

Clothes made of synthetic fibres such as nylon do not absorb moisture and can be hazardous. They may also cause the patient to slide down the bed, increasing the risk of tissue damage from shear. Bedding should be relatively free from wrinkles. Tight bedding should also be avoided as this may restrict movement, in particular over the feet where heels would be at risk. Bed cradles can be used to keep bed linen away from feet. Where specialist bed systems are used tight linen can substantially reduce their effectiveness.

## Sleep and Rest

Sleep deprivation and restlessness are potential predisposing factors in the development of pressure sores. Studies have shown that tissue renewal is greatest at rest and during sleep (for example, Oswald and Adam, 1984). Consideration for adequate rest and sleep is, therefore, important when planning a patient's care. Care and treatment should only be given overnight where necessary and planned so as to allow maximum periods of time where the patient is undisturbed. Noise levels must be kept to a minimum so as to allow for rest and sleep. If specialist pressure-relieving equipment is indicated, the type of system selected should be comfortable and quiet so as to allow for rest and sleep. Some specialist beds reduce the need for repositioning and hence the number of times that a patient is disturbed. Repositioning is important to prevent joint stiffness and may be a necessary component in other aspects of the patient's care and treatment, for example chest drainage. However, these systems are particularly useful where frequent repositioning is required in order to prevent pressure sores. Medication to aid sleep may be considered, however caution should be exercised as these medications can reduce sensation and movement. The use of medication to aid sleep should, therefore, be carefully considered as the therapeutic value may not equate with the potential adverse effects.

## Medication

Many drugs can increase an individual's susceptibility to the development of pressure sores.

Tranquillisers, sedatives and opiates can reduce an individual's sensation and level of mobility. Steroids have an anti-inflammatory effect and may, therefore, impair the inflammatory stage of the healing process. Inflammation is part of the restorative process in tissue damage, whereby there is increased blood flow to the area and an influx of white blood cells. Steroids also reduce protein synthesis, fibroblast and epithelial proliferation rates (Dealey, 1991), which reduces tissue quality. Cytotoxic drugs act to destroy rapidly dividing malignant cells, however they also destroy normal cells and impair the healing process.

## Cardiovascular and Respiratory Function

Any condition that reduces the quantity or quality of tissue blood supply will potentiate the likelihood of pressure sore development. It is well documented that patients with cardiovascular problems are predisposed to pressure sores. Cardiac disorders, peripheral vascular disease, anaemia and other circulatory disorders are potent predisposing factors. Several authors recommend maintaining the haemo-globin level at 12.5 g/dl, for example, Vasile and Chaitin, 1972, who found that the haemoglobin level was of critical importance in the prognosis of patients with pressure sores. They reported an average haemoglobin level of 12.7 g/dl in the surviving group as opposed to an average of 9.4 g/dl in those who died. Adequate cardiac output to maintain a healthy perfusion of peripheral tissue is essential. Oedema may compromise metabolite exchange and, additionally, arteriosclerotic disease may reduce the flow of blood to the tissues. Many authors have emphasised that reduced blood flow can be an important factor in pressure sore development. Barton (1977) considered the first 48 hours following an episode of shock as being especially hazardous.

Smoking is another factor related to pressure sore development. Barton (1977) found pressure sores on the heels of smokers to be four times more likely than for non-smokers. It seems that the vascular effects of smoking are the most likely explanation, i.e. nicotine causes vasoconstriction.

Any respiratory disease that leads to reduced blood oxygen content will predispose to the development of pressure sores by tissue hypoxia. However, appropriate treatment of cardiovascular, periph-eral vascular and respiratory problems can greatly increase a patient's ability to resist tissue damage. Maintenance of good cardiac output, the reduction of oedema and correction of anaemia are particularly important.

## Neurological Disease

The link between neurological disease and the development of pres-sure sores is well recognised (for example, Bader, 1990; David et al., 1983). Neurological disease may alter appreciation of pain and a reduction in mobility alters response to stimuli, for example continu-ous pressure. The 'trophic' theory of pressure sore development proposes that damage to the nerve supply of a tissue deprives it of a nutritive element (as yet unrecognised) and suggests that this can result in a predisposition to tissue damage. Other research does not favour the trophic theory (Whimster, 1976). A more obvious link is the effect of neurological impairment on mobility and sensation, e.g. paraplegia, multiple sclerosis. Epidural anaesthesia or analgesia also causes an enforced, but temporary, reduction in sensation and/or mobility. Individuals receiving epidural anaesthesia or analgesia require special consideration for pressure sore prevention, particularly at the sacrum, even if no other predisposing factors have been identified.

## Metabolic Disorders

The body's reaction to infection is to raise the metabolic rate, particularly its demand for oxygen, which renders an individual more vulnerable to tissue damage. Severe systemic infections cause the body's protein pool to be depleted and the immune system may be overworked and unable to counteract local skin damage as well as systemic infection. Pyrexia increases the metabolic rate, in particular the demand for oxygen, which endangers ischaemic areas. Severe infection can also cause nutritional disturbances and local bacteria increase the demand on local metabolism by both their own requirements and the response of the body's defence mechanism. If the temperature of tissues that are under load is raised, their metabolic rate and oxygen consumption are increased, while capillary blood flow is reduced. This brings an increased risk of cellular death. Some support surfaces can cause an increase in tissue temperature through insulation. Increased temperature also causes sweating, which alters skin integrity through maceration.

The vascular effects of diabetes mellitus, liver enzyme insufficiency and raised blood urea may also lead to increased susceptibility to tissue damage.

## Age

The integrity of the skin is challenged by the ageing process, which causes reduction in skin elasticity, loss of subcutaneous fat, a decrease in cell proliferation and collagen disposition, and a degree of muscle atrophy. The elderly may also have multiple pathology, which also increases their vulnerability to tissue damage.

## Conclusion

The preventative management of pressure sores should focus on controlling or alleviating identified predisposing factors in addition to minimising exposure to the precipitating factors of pressure, shear and friction. The patient's plan of care may require multidisciplinary collaboration and agreement reached in relation to the required care and treatments from each professional group.

# Chapter 9:
# Equipment Guide

- standard foam mattresses
- static mattress overlays
- dynamic mattress overlays and specialist bed systems
- seating
- miscellaneous aids

The purpose of this chapter is to provide guidance in the selection and use of equipment for pressure sore prevention. It is not intended to be an exhaustive guide and refers to generic types of equipment and their relative merits as opposed to specific company products.

Equipment can be expensive and for this reason a rational decision-making framework should be used to target resources to identified areas on the basis of need.

There should be a multidisciplinary approach in the selection of equipment for patients, based on a comprehensive assessment that aims to identify factors which render the patient at risk of developing pressure sores. Surfaces on which a patient is placed are particularly important and should be carefully considered.

All equipment needs to be suitable for the purpose intended, well maintained in a safe and reliable condition and be readily available for use.

## Characteristics of the Ideal Patient Bed

The ideal patient support system:

1. distributes pressure evenly, or provides frequent relief of pressure, or provides constant low pressure
2. conforms to body weight

3.    minimises friction and shearing forces
4.    provides a well ventilated, comfortable surface that does not
      unduly restrict movement
5.    maintains skin at a constant optimal temperature
6.    is acceptable to the patient
7.    does not impede care interventions, and can quickly provide a
      hard surface for resuscitation procedures
8.    is easily cleaned and maintained
9.    is easily operated by both carers and patient
10.   should have the following features:
         height adjustment;
         tilt facility;
         sufficient clearance for hoist, if necessary;
         be mobile, with efficient brakes.

(See Torrance, 1983.)

# Standard Foam Mattresses

### Guidelines for Mattress Selection

Although a hospital bed mattress may seem a minor component in
comparison with other more sophisticated equipment involved in
pressure sore prevention, judicious selection can make a significant
difference in reducing the incidence of pressure sores.

### *Mattress Effectiveness*

A range of foam mattresses have been extensively evaluated for their
effectiveness by the Department of Health (1993b), with particular
regard to their pressure reduction properties. The mattresses
selected for evaluation included the standard NHS contract foam
mattress and a number of alternative foam mattresses. The issue of
tissue interface pressure was central to this study. Tissue interface
pressure refers to the external pressure to which tissues are exposed
by any surface in contact with them. Therefore, the lower the interface pressure the lower the pressure on the tissue capillaries. The
standard NHS contract foam mattresses were found to produce
interface pressures of approximately 130 mmHg. Tissue interface
pressure of approximately 20 mmHg can be sufficient to cause capillary occlusion in a healthy individual (Landis, 1930). All the alternative foam mattresses showed significant reduction in interface
pressures relative to that of the standard NHS contract mattress. The
report concluded that the interface pressures encountered on standard NHS contract mattresses make them unsuitable for anyone at

any risk of developing pressure sores, and that they do not provide a comfortable surface to lie on.

Manufacturers information on the effectiveness of their mattresses is often limited (Department of Health, 1993b; Rithalia, 1993; Young, 1990). Caution should be taken when interpreting mattress effectiveness through manufacturers claims, as they are often made on the basis of inadequate, invalid and unreliable data.

### Mattress Durability

Even the best mattress will be of little clinical use if it is unable to stand up to the rigours of use on a ward. It is important therefore that a mattress is made of a good quality foam. A good quality foam has the ability to return to its original shape once body weight has been removed. Because of its fine cell structure, polyurethane foam has become the preferred support surface medium. The foam density is the key indication of its quality. This is defined as the weight of the foam per unit volume — often kilograms per cubic metre ($kg/m^3$). A high-density foam is more expensive but it retains its support properties for longer. The standard NHS contract mattress is made from a single block of polyether foam, and has a density of 39–42 $kg/m^3$ (Department of Health, 1993b). Most alternative mattresses are made from multiple layers of polyurethane foam which vary in density from 33 to 90 $kg/m^3$ (Department of Health, 1993b).

In the Department of Health comparative evaluation of foam mattresses (1993b), all mattresses tested appeared to dent under the area of maximum weight and contact after only a short period of time. With the standard NHS contract mattress this denting was to such an extent that the base of the bed could be felt when a hand compression test was applied — a phenomenon described as 'bottoming-out'. The denting in all other mattresses appeared to resolve once the weight was removed, by either turning the mattress or leaving it unoccupied for a short period. In conclusion, the report questions the durability of the standard NHS contract mattress. Most manufacturers give an estimate of the life of their mattresses, and some provide a guarantee. The Department of Health (1993b) suggests that it is vitally important, in light of the foam-denting phenomenon, to turn mattresses at least weekly. It is also important to employ a mattress replacement policy so that mattresses are checked regularly for their suitability and are replaced when found to be no longer suitable for use.

### Mattress Suitability

It is important to consider whether a mattress will be suitable for the application to which you wish to put it. The standard NHS contract mattress is not recommended for use with anyone who is at any risk of developing pressure sores (Department of Health, 1993b). Alternative foam mattresses are suitable for patients who are 'at risk' of developing pressure sores, but who are not considered to be in sufficient danger to warrant using a specialist pressure-relieving system. Regular patient risk assessment is necessary to ensure that the mattress will provide the required degree of protection. (See chapter 7 entitled Risk Assessment and chapter 8, Preventative Management.)

Accident & Emergency, X-ray, Operating Theatre and other specialist departments must give consideration to the special needs of patients at risk of developing pressure sores, and develop their own systems of management to deal with them. Replacement trolley mattresses are available which are designed to provide a greater degree of pressure relief than standard trolley mattresses, and mattress overlays are also available.

### Mattress Covers

A Department of Health study (1993b) highlighted the difference that the covering material can make to the pressure-reducing properties of a mattress. The standard NHS contract mattress is supplied with a non-stretch, polyvinyl chloride-coated nylon cover (usually with a pink marble effect). The application of a one-way stretch material cover to this mattress resulted in a significant improvement in tissue interface pressures. The application of a heavy-duty vinyl cover to this mattress resulted an extremely high interface pressure, and was therefore not recommended for use.

Essential qualities of a mattress cover:

> waterproof
> water vapour permeable
> fire retardant to BS 6807
> stretch material
> durable material
> tight fitting and wrinkle-free on mattress to BS 5224 (Part 4)

### Mattress Care and Maintenance

### Turning

A Department of Health study (1993b) highlighted the phenomenon of foam denting (bottoming-out) at areas of maximum weight and contact. This problem was found to resolve once the weight was removed, by either turning the mattress or leaving it unoccupied for a short period. In order to minimise this effect, and so minimise tissue interface pressures, and in order to prolong the life expectancy of the mattress, it is very important to turn the mattress on a regular basis, e.g. weekly or between patients, whichever is the more frequent. Some mattresses can be purchased with turning clocks printed on the cover. In the absence of a preprinted turning regimen mattresses should be marked with one (Figure 9.1).

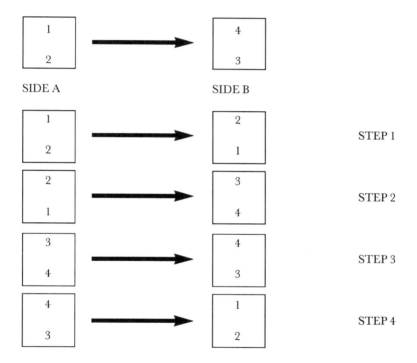

**Figure 9.1** Mattress turning regimen

### *Cleaning*

Manufacturers instructions should always be adhered to, with consideration for local infection control policy requirements. An infection control nurse should be contacted for further advice.

Generally, the following guidelines are recommended for use between patients:

- wash with warm water and neutral detergent
- in cases of soiling, the following is recommended:
  Milton disinfectant *then* warm water and neutral detergent
  Note: phenolics should never be used, and disinfectants should always be washed off after their use in order to avoid mattress cover breakdown.
    always allow the mattress to dry thoroughly
    all bed bases should be either corrugated or mesh in order to avoid mattress condensation problems.

## Mattress Replacement Policy

All mattresses should be marked with their date of issue on supply to clinical areas and both the mattresses and their covers must be checked for their suitability every 6 months. A mattress replacement strategy should be in place in each clinical area, i.e. managers must forward plan and budget for mattress replacement.

### Criteria for the Assessment of Mattress Covers

The absence of any of the following characteristics requires the mattress cover to be replaced:

- Water resistance
  A Department of Health regulation — absence of water resistance presents an infection hazard.
  *Water penetration test:* Undo zip of mattress cover and place sheet of absorbent tissue between the cover and the mattress foam. Using a fist, indent the mattress to form a shallow well and pour approximately half a cup of water into the well. Agitate the water for approximately 1 minute in order to increase its contact with the surface of the mattress, and then mop the water up. Inspect the tissue for water marking. Repeat this procedure on the reverse side of the mattress.
- Integrity
  Worn areas and tears allow moisture and dirt to penetrate to the mattress foam and represent an infection hazard.
- Stretch material
  The Department of Health (1993b) reported that non-stretch covers caused high tissue interface pressures and were therefore not recommended for use.

Note: the absence of a water-resistant and/or intact mattress cover may require the whole mattress to be replaced.

**Criteria for the Assessment of Mattress Foams**

- Effectiveness
  *Hand compression test:*
  Place both hands on the mattress and press down using your full body weight. Repeat for the entire length of the mattress. Note any variation in the density of the foam, including whether the base of the bed can be felt through the foam — a phenomenon called 'grounding' or bottoming-out.
  Note: grounding or bottoming-out significantly increases the risk of pressure sore formation. The mattress should be replaced immediately.
- Depth of foam
  A Department of Health regulation requires a mattress to be at least 130 mm in depth. This does not apply to trolley mattresses.
- Condition of mattress foam
  Unzip the mattress cover and inspect the foam for signs of staining, odour, moisture or crumbling. Any of these characteristics require the foam to be replaced.

# Summary points

- Standard NHS contract mattresses are unsuitable for anyone at any risk of developing sores (Department of Health, 1993b)
- Mattress covers significantly affect the pressure-relieving properties of a mattress (Department of Health, 1993b)
- Caution should be taken when interpreting mattress effectiveness from manufacturer claims
- Mattresses must be marked with the date of issue on supply to a clinical area
- Mattresses must be turned weekly or between patients (whichever is the more frequent) to minimise the effects of foam denting
- Mattresses should be cleaned between patients or weekly
- Mattress covers and foams must be assessed every 6 months for their suitability
- A mattress replacement policy should operate in every clinical area

## Static Mattress Overlays

A range of static mattress overlays have recently been evaluated by the Department of Health (1994), with particular regard to their pressure-reducing properties. This study does not claim to be exhaustive, as there is an enormous range of products of this type available, however some of the most commonly used types of static mattress overlays were evaluated.

The study included four categories of static mattress overlay:

*   fibre-filled overlays
*   foam overlays
*   air-filled overlays
*   fleece overlays

The issue of tissue interface pressure was central to this study. Tissue interface pressure refers to the external pressure to which tissues are exposed by any surface in contact with them. The lower the interface pressure, the lower the pressure on the tissue capillaries. Tissue interface pressure of approximately 20 mmHg can be sufficient to cause capillary occlusion in a healthy individual (Landis, 1930). The results of the tissue interface pressure, which are outlined below, are relative to the familiar standard NHS contract mattress with which average tissue interface pressures measured are approximately 130 mmHg, depending on the site evaluated (Department of Health, 1993b). Tissue interface pressures were measured over the sacrum, trochanter and heels of elderly volunteers.

### Fibre-filled Overlays

When new, all the fibre-filled overlays tested gave quite good interface pressure reduction over all three sites. There was little difference between the pressure reduction measurements obtained on all of the overlays tested. When these overlays were retested after 6 months of clinical use a different pattern emerged. All of the overlays gave significantly less pressure reduction than when new. The collective deterioration seen after 6 months of clinical use was not caused by laundering as most overlays were not washed during this period — the waterproof covers were cleaned between patients by nursing staff. The statistically significant reduction in their effectiveness after only 6 months of use suggests that they provide less pressure reduction than the better standard foam mattresses. There were two fibre-filled overlays that did not have all-enclosing waterproof covers, and which were therefore subjected to washing and drying cycles according to the protocol specified by the manufacturers. The interface pressures were retested after each laundering episode. No statistically significant difference was noted in the interface pressure readings after laundering. It is recognised however that hospital laundering services may not always follow manufacturers instructions, which may influence the effectiveness of the overlay in relation to its pressure-reducing properties.

### Clinical Evaluation

Those fibre-filled overlays with all-enclosing waterproof covers were considered by the clinical users in the evaluation to be advantageous as this allowed cleaning to take place on the ward, preventing the need for their removal from the ward and clinical use. All the overlays evaluated were found to give a good degree of comfort and were acceptable to all users. However, in some instances they were found to impede mobilisation on and off the bed. Some degree of flattening occurred under the areas of maximum load with all the fibre-filled overlays whilst in use.

### Guidelines for Use

Because of the dramatic deterioration in effectiveness in their first 6 months of clinical use, without laundering, fibre-filled overlays are recommended only for patients at low risk of developing pressure sores or for comfort purposes. These overlays can be useful in reducing the effects of shear and friction, and for minimising skin maceration from excess moisture accumulation.

## Foam Overlays

The interface pressure-reducing properties of the foam overlays when new were not as good as the best fibre-filled overlays when new. However, after 6 months of clinical use their properties were much less changed than those of all the fibre-filled overlays after 6 months of clinical use. This retained effectiveness, combined with their relatively low cost, makes them an attractive option. The foam did appear to soften up slightly over the areas of maximum load, however this did not unduly affect their pressure-relieving characteristics.

### Clinical Evaluation

These were found by the users to provide a good degree of support and comfort. They were found not to impede patient mobilisation on and off the bed as much as other overlays tested.

*Guidelines for Use*

These foam overlays are recommended for use with patients at low to medium risk of developing pressure sores. Foam overlays can however cause a rise in tissue temperature through insulation. If the temperature of tissues which are under load is raised, their metabolic rate and oxygen consumption requirements are increased, whilst the capillary blood flow is reduced. This brings an increased risk of cellular death. Some foam overlays also increase the likelihood of tissue maceration through excess skin moisture. They should therefore ideally have moisture-permeable covers.

**Air-filled Overlays**

The air-filled overlays gave the best interface pressure readings of all those overlays evaluated in the study. The air-filled overlays give the same interface pressure readings after 6 months of clinical use provided that they are correctly inflated.

*Clinical Evaluation*

These overlays were found to be comfortable by the users, although some users found that the overlays made it difficult to get on and off the bed. There was however resistance by nursing staff to using them because of the inflation procedure required for each patient using the overlays. These overlays need to be monitored carefully for puncture.

*Guidelines for Use*

Air-filled overlays are recommended for use with patients at medium risk of developing pressure sores. The overlays evaluated were low-profile, static mattresses and therefore not recommended for use with patients at greater risk of developing pressure sores.

**Fleece Overlays**

Two fleeces were evaluated — one 100% polyester and one 100% wool. The fleeces gave best pressure reduction when used for heels, however they were not considered to be a satisfactory means of pressure reduction in comparison with that of other overlays. There was a significant reduction in interface pressure reduction between both fleeces when new and when 6 months old, however the synthetic fleece became more matted than the wool fleece.

*Guidelines for Use*

Fleeces should be regarded primarily as comfort aids. Fleeces do however provide some protection from the effects of shear and friction, and can reduce skin maceration from excess moisture. Marchand and Lidowski (1993) found that wool fleeces were more effective in reducing the effects of friction and shear than synthetic fleeces due to the natural oils which create a slick surface, and their moisture absorption properties which help to maintain proper hydration of the epidermis. Fleeces can however be a potential reservoir for infection. They should not be used on specialist bed or seat systems as they are likely to increase interface pressures.

## Dynamic Mattress Overlays and Specialist Bed Systems

A large range of dynamic mattress overlays and specialist bed systems are available from a variety of suppliers. In the main these products have been poorly evaluated. For example, trials on constant low-pressure support systems were found to be flawed in both research design and statistical evaluation (Bliss and Thomas, 1993).

Indeed, it is evident that much of the available literature is produced by the suppliers themselves and is rarely underpinned with rigorous scientific research. It should also be noted that such studies have not, as yet, provided a comprehensive comparative guide to the selection of dynamic mattress overlays and specialist bed systems. This is perhaps because in the past suppliers have been unwilling to allow their products to be comparatively evaluated in a properly conducted research trial.

### Equipment Selection

The most effective way of selecting a dynamic mattress overlay or specialist bed system is to consider the objectives for its use. With the aid of suppliers' literature these objectives can then be matched with the functionality of the equipment available (see objectives for equipment use). An additional guide to decision making, outlining some of the clinical facts that should be taken into consideration, can be found in Table 9.1. Any decision should always be made in conjunction with an up-to-date risk assessment score, advice from the company nurse representative and, of course, in the light of clinical judgement of relevant healthcare professionals.

**Table 9.1** Decision-making guide for the selection of pressure-relieving equipment[1]

| Risk factors | No risk/minimal risk | Low risk | At risk/compromised | Compromised/tissue breakdown | Compromised/extensive tissue breakdown | Complications of immobility |
|---|---|---|---|---|---|---|
| **Skin integrity** | Intact skin | Small reddened areas on bony prominences that blanch/may have skin sensitivities | Reddened areas but skin intact | One or more areas of superficial breakdown. Some areas may have full involvement. Wound care is necessary | One or more areas of full-thickness and/or deep tissue damage. Needs improved cutaneous circulation | Any of previous categories |
| **Mobility** | Ambulatory/short hospital stay anticipated | Limited mobility; may require assistance with turning and/or walking | Limited mobility | Limited mobility | Limited mobility | Severely limited mobility or immobile |
| **Nutrition** | Adequate nutritional status | Adequate nutritional status | Inadequate oral intake; questionable nutritional status | Malnourished | Malnourished | Any of previous categories |
| **Continence** | Continent | Continent or indwelling urinary catheter | Frequent or total incontinence; no urinary catheter | Incontinent | Incontinent | Any of previous categories |
| **Sensory factors** | Normal | Normal | May have decreased sensation | Altered | Altered | Any of previous categories |
| **Mental status** | Normal | Normal | May be receiving sedatives, narcotics, barbiturates, psychotropic medication | Altered | Altered | Any of previous categories |
| **Weight** | Normal | Normal | May be over or under weight | May be over or under weight | Altered | Any of previous categories |
| **Suggestions for support surface** | Good quality standard foam mattress | Static mattress overlay and frequent risk reassessment | Dynamic mattress overlay | Specialist pressure-relieving system | Air fluidised surface | Ask for specific advice from company representative |

[1] This guide should be used in conjunction with clinical judgement, a risk assessment score and advice from a company representative

## Objectives for Equipment Use

The following factors should be taken into consideration when trying to match treatment objectives against equipment functionality:

- prevention of skin trauma caused by pressure, friction and shear forces when a turning schedule is not effective, appropriate or possible
- relief of pain and the promotion of comfort, rest and sleep by reducing patient handling
- provision of an ideal external wound-healing environment for pressure sores, traumatic wounds, plastic surgery and burns
- minimisation of maceration in cases of incontinence, exuding wounds and excessive sweating
- regulation of body temperature in cases of hypo- or hyperthermia, peripheral shutdown, or for the effects of catabolism and protein sparing
- facilitation of nursing and medical procedures

## Relationship with Equipment Suppliers

Most hospitals and community units will have contracts with leading suppliers of dynamic mattress overlays and specialist bed systems. A mutually beneficial, professional relationship with these suppliers and in particular with the nurse representatives should be established. The aim of this relationship is to work in partnership, thus ensuring the best possible service for patients.

## Ordering Rental Equipment

Equipment should be ordered in accordance with directorate, ward or department policies for financial expenditure. If in doubt, advice should be sought from the relevant manager.

# Seating

Seating provided in the hospital setting is often inappropriate for the user (Gebhardt and Bliss, 1994; Lowry, 1992). In addition to the importance of suitable seating in wards, there is an equal need to consider the requirements of patients attending other hospital departments.

Encouraging patients to sit in chairs as opposed to remaining in bed during the day, so-called 'chair nursing', is widely thought to prevent pressure sores and other complications associated with bedrest, such as venous thrombosis, chest infection, urinary tract infection and constipation (Middleton, 1983; Pritchard and David, 1984; Wilson, 1985). Findings in a recent study (Gebhardt and Bliss, 1994) do not support this theory. The results suggest that the development of pressure sores is strongly correlated with the length of individual periods of time spent sitting. Those patients whose 'chair nursing' was restricted to less than 2 hours per session, compared with similar patients who sat for longer periods, suffered fewer chest infections, were less constipated and appeared less fatigued and more active and motivated. They also mobilised earlier than patients who experienced 'chair nursing'. Patients should be encouraged to get in and out of bed as frequently as they wish, but with caution exercised in relation to the length of time spent sitting in any one session. Ideally, sitting should involve other activities, for example, a meal, watching television, seeing visitors or reading. The first sitting period should be for no longer than 30 minutes without the skin being inspected for tolerance. If no marking occurs, this sitting time can be gradually increased but should not exceed 2 hours (Gebhardt and Bliss, 1994).

**Principles of Good Seating**

A good comfortable position should not cause overstrain of any particular group of muscles, and should allow an individual to maintain a position without undue effort. Whether standing or sitting, the key to a good posture is the position of the pelvis. This will not only determine skeletal posture, but also flexibility and mobility, and therefore function in that position. Poor sitting posture and an ill-fitting seating system will result in pain and discomfort from muscular and skeletal strain, with increased risk of developing pressure sores and contractures. It will also have an effect on the function of the inner organs as well as the mental state. Imagine the difference in effect on a person's mental state with an upright posture compared with that of an individual in a slumped posture.

For any seating system to be successful it is important that the user and carers are well informed about the principles of good posture, the seating system itself, its potential for adjustment and its potential hazards. Poor posture is often the result of a bad habit. Advice about how to correct posture will go a long way in preventing otherwise devastating effects.

A decision-making guide for the selection of seating can be found at the end of this chapter (see Table 9.2).

**Chairs**

A good chair must be comfortable, support the patient in a good posture and allow the individual to sit down in it and stand up from it easily. A lot of chairs tend to be low and are therefore unsuitable for anyone with weak or painful lower limbs. Chairs can also be deep and slanted at the back, therefore providing little lumbar support.

### Chair Height

When the patient is sitting, their hips, knees and ankles should ideally be at right angles to each other. With adults, this usually means that a chair of at least 45 cm (18 inches) high is required. Chairs can be raised by putting them on blocks, which may be preferable to adding an extra cushion as this will often make the chair too soft to rise from, or the armrest too low.

### Chair Depth

The chair should support the patient's thighs and allow his or her bottom to reach the back of the chair leaving a gap of 5–8 cm (2–3 inches) between the front of the chair and the back of the knees.

### Chair Width

A chair must be roomy enough to allow the patient to move about a little to relieve pressure on one part of their body, whilst also allowing the armrests to be used in aiding standing and sitting.

### Chair Firmness

The chair should be firm yet comfortable, as firm seats are much easier to get out of than soft ones. Special cushions are available for use with patients at varying risk of developing pressure sores.

### Chair Back

The back of the chair should be high enough to support the patient's head and should have a lumbar curve to support the back.

### Chair Armrest

The armrest should come far enough forward to provide good leverage for standing up but not so far forward as to make the chair unstable.

## Wheelchairs

A well chosen wheelchair should maximise the user's mobility, independence, comfort and confidence. The basic requirements are for a stable, adjustable seat, which is easy to use and manoeuvre, by both the disabled person and any helpers, and which is robust.

There is a very wide range of wheelchairs available and each person's needs and preferences differ. It is important therefore to take care in choosing the most appropriate model. Relatively minor modifications in design, components and appearance can have a major impact on the performance of the chair and on the user's satisfaction. Wheelchairs should be chosen with the advice of a therapist who is familiar with the types of wheelchair available. Careful evaluation is required before a wheelchair is chosen to meet the user's personal preferences, skills, life style as well as a particular medical condition. A selection should only be made after considering all the options and trying out a number of different models. More than one chair may be required to fulfil all requirements, e.g. for travel, work, sports, and indoor and outdoor use.

The principal measurements required for selecting a wheelchair are those of the user, the wheelchair, the height and strength of any carer, and also consideration for where the chair is to be used. The measurements required of the user are:

- the distance from the seat to the level of the shoulders when sitting
- the distance from the back of the buttocks to behind the knees
- the distance from behind the knees to the heels
- the distance from the seat to the forearms with the elbows flexed
- weight
- relative strength in manoeuvring a chair

Ideally, when sitting the individual's hips, knees and ankle joints should be at right angles to each other. The backrest should be sufficiently high to provide mid-scapula support, although people with weak trunks will require more support. The armrest should allow the arms to rest at right angles without hunching the shoulders. The chair should be designed to take the patient's weight. For individuals who are able to self-propel the chair the wheels should be within easy reach without having to stretch, and for those who use controls these should also be within easy reach on the armrest.

## Seat Cushions

The function of a cushion is to reduce pressure and shear forces and thus reduce the likelihood of tissue damage. It should also provide comfort and a support for the user. Seat cushions rarely result in ischial pressure readings below the capillary blood pressure as the surface area bearing the upper body weight is very small; over 50% of the body weight is supported on 8% of the sitting area at or near the ischial tuberosities (Staas and Cioschi, 1991). Advice should be sought from an occupational therapist when choosing a pressure-relieving cushion as it will alter the effectiveness of the backrest, armrest and seat height, and the position of the person in the chair. There is little available comparative evaluative research in relation to seat cushions.

### Fibre-filled Cushions

These cushions are generally recommended for patients with only a low risk of developing pressure sores, although there is little research available on their effect on interface pressure. A study of the effectiveness of fibre-filled mattress overlays has recently been published (Department of Health, 1994), which indicates that they can achieve good reductions in tissue interface pressures; however, they were found to deteriorate in effectiveness rapidly in their first 6 months of clinical use, without laundering, such that they were recommended only for patients of low risk or for comfort purposes. They can be useful in preventing the effects of shear and friction, and for minimising skin maceration from excess moisture accumulation.

### Foam Cushions

Foam cushions are available in different thicknesses, shapes and types of foam. There are many proprietary alternatives. The foam density is the key indicator of a good quality product. A high-density foam is more expensive but will retain its support properties for longer. Polyurethane foam is commonly used because it is lightweight and cheap, but the density of the foam is the key indicator of its usefulness. Foams of different densities also allow for different weights of user. Sometimes, the foam block will have a divided surface, often resembling that of an 'egg box'.

Foam cushions are usually recommended for patients at low to medium risk of developing pressure sores, however this will vary according to the different composition of the cushions. Foam cushions also insulate and cause tissue temperatures to rise. If the temperature of tissues that are under load is raised, their metabolic rate and oxygen consumption requirements are increased, whilst the capillary blood flow may be reduced. This brings an increased risk of cellular death.

Some foam cushions also increase the likelihood of tissue maceration through excess skin moisture. They should ideally therefore have moisture-permeable covers. All foam cushions require regular evaluation of their durability as some only have an effective life of 6 months.

### Air-filled Cushions

Air-filled cushions consist of rows of inflatable cells where the pressure is adjusted appropriately for each individual patient. Cushions of this type can be active or static.

The active cushions of this type are connected to a pump that operates by alternately inflating and deflating the air cells so as to change the interface pressures experienced at frequent intervals. This type of air-filled cushion is generally recommended for patients at a medium to high risk of developing pressures sores.

The static cushions of this type comprise those of low and high profile; low profile is recommended for patients at medium to high risk of developing pressure sores, and the high profile for patients at very high risk of developing pressure sores. These types of cushions offer the best pressure relief on the market if appropriately used (Bar, 1991), but can be highly detrimental if incorrectly used. Both under- and over-inflation of the air cells will result in increased tissue interface pressures. Best effects are obtained by sitting directly on the cushion, therefore a cover should be avoided.

### *Fleeces*

Most literature available suggests that whilst these cushions do provide a degree of pressure reduction, this is only sufficient to make them suitable for patients at low risk of developing pressure sores. It is suggested that their prime use is for comfort purposes, to reduce friction or shear, or to reduce skin maceration from excess moisture. They should not be used on specialist seat systems as they are likely to increase interface pressures. A recent study (Department of Health, 1994) has indicated that there is no significant difference in effectiveness between wool and polyester fleeces, however polyester fleece was more susceptible to becoming matted. Both require careful laundering. Marchand and Lidowski (1993) found that wool fleece was more effective in reducing the effects of friction and shear than polyester fleece due to the natural oils which create a slick surface, and its moisture absorption properties which help to maintain proper hydration of the epidermis. Fleeces can be a potential reservoir for infection.

### *Ring Cushions*

Ring cushions can be either foam or air-filled. They are shaped like a doughnut, with a hole in the centre of a circular cushion. Various research suggests that lymphatic drainage and circulation are adversely affected by the use of these cushions. There is a general consensus of opinion that they are unsuitable and potentially harmful. These cushions are therefore not recommended for use.

**Table 9.2** Decision-making guide for the selection of seating products

| Low risk/comfort aids | Fibre-filled cushions<br>Fleeces<br>Foam cushions |
|---|---|
| Medium risk | Foam cushions<br>Low-profile static air-filled cushions<br>Active air-filled cushions |
| High risk | Low-profile static air-filled cushions<br>High-profile static air-filled cushions<br>Active air-filled cushions |
| Very high risk | High-profile static air-filled cushions |

# Miscellaneous aids

### Pads and Booties

Heel and elbow pads can provide protection from shear and friction damage, but do not offer advantages in terms of pressure relief.

### Water-filled Gloves

Lockyer-Stevens (1993) found that water-filled gloves placed under a patient's heels provide insufficient pressure relief to prevent pressure sores. Although the practice of using water-filled gloves is widespread, there is no evidence to support it. These can also be uncomfortable and irritating for the patient.

### Bath Cushions

There are cushions available for use in the bath, designed so as not to float! They are suitable for use with any patient who is at risk of pressure sores whilst in the bath.

### Toilet/Commode/Hoist Cushions

These cushions are shaped to fit most toilets, commodes and hoists, and are usually attached using Velcro strips. They are suitable for use with any patient who is at risk of pressure sores whilst using a toilet, commode or hoist.

# Chapter 10:
# Education

## Staff Education

It could be argued that education is the single most effective way of reducing the incidence of pressure sores. Dealey (1992b) found that the introduction of an educational programme alone resulted in a decrease in annual pressure sore prevalence rates from 13.9% to 5.6%.

A wide range of staff require education in relation to pressure sore prevention, including medical practitioners, nurses, healthcare assistants, managers, dieticians, therapists, pharmacists, supplies officers, and others. Managers have a key responsibility both for considering priorities and in providing staff with the appropriate opportunities for education and training. There are several educational packages available.

*Videos:*

*   'Focus on Pressure Sores'
    The Tissue Viability Society
    Wessex Rehabilitation Association
    Salisbury District Hospital
    Salisbury
    Wiltshire SP2 8BJ
    Telephone: 01722 336262

*   'A Sore Point — Managing the Stages of Pressure Sores'
    Healthcare
    2 Stucley Place
    Camden Lock
    London NW1 8NS
    Telephone: 0171 267 8757

- 'Pressure Sores — the Hidden Epidemic'
  Concord Video & Film Council
  201 Felixstowe Road
  Ipswich
  IP3 9BH
  Telephone: 01473 715754

*Study days:*

The Tissue Viability Society will arrange free study days anywhere in the country on request. These events can be run in the workplace and staff have the choice of attending either the morning or afternoon session.

## Patient Education

Patients are responsible for furthering their own health gain and avoiding the deterioration of their health status, in so far as they have the knowledge and the capability to do so. Patients are dependent on the multidisciplinary team to provide them with information about their condition and training in the practicalities of helping themselves.

It is important to involve patients in the planning of their treatment and care in order to provide the opportunity for them to influence the treatment and care that they receive. The rationale for pressure sore prevention interventions should, whenever possible, be discussed with the patient and verbal consent and cooperation obtained. Aspects of self-care for pressure sore prevention should be taught and the patient's progress with self-care aspects reviewed regularly.

The Department of Health have published a booklet for patients entitled 'Your Guide to Pressure Sores' which is available by telephoning the Health Literature Line on 0800 555777.

The Tissue Viability Society have published a patient booklet entitled 'Skin Care — Your Guide to the Prevention and Treatment of Pressure Sores'. It is available from:

The Tissue Viability Society
Wessex Rehabilitation Association
Salisbury District Hospital
Salisbury
Wiltshire
SP2 8BJ
Telephone: 01722 336262

## Action Points

Information and education should be provided for patients and carers in relation to the following:

- What a pressure sore is and the implication of pressure sore development
- Risks known to increase pressure sore development
- How patients can practically help themselves to prevent the development of pressure sores, including information on mobility, positioning in bed and chairs, skin care, nutrition and hydration
- How to recognise the early signs of skin damage, and who to tell if skin damage is noticed
- Where to get further information

# Chapter 11: Audit

A systematic approach to the evaluation of a pressure sore prevention strategy requires the collection of data which accurately describe the nature of the problem of pressure sores within a hospital or community unit.

This chapter describes a framework for the audit of pressure sores, which is loosely based on the considerations for audit as described by Lockyer-Stevens (1994) (Table 11.1). At the end of this chapter there are two examples of Standards of Care related to pressure sore prevention, as used at Chelsea & Westminster Hospital, London.

**Table 11.1** Considerations for effective audit

| |
|---|
| • How frequently to audit |
| • Method of audit |
| • Areas to be included in audit |
| • Classification of pressure sores |
| • Methods of data collection |
| • Data analysis |
| • Data reporting |

## How Frequently to Audit

The duration or frequency of data collection may range from continuous surveillance to once or twice a year. Prevalence surveys involve data collection on an intermittent rather than continuous basis. By taking a cross-sectional sample of the hospital population (that is all patients who are in hospital on the day of audit), prevalence data indicate the number of patients with a pressure sore in relation to the total number of patients, and may be collected annually, 6 monthly or monthly.

Incidence surveillance involves continuous data collection on the number of patients who either have or develop pressure sores.

## Method of Audit

The consensus view on the relative merits of the two audit methods, as described here, is that incidence data are preferable to prevalence data. This view is summarised by Cullum and Shakespeare (1994), who state that prevalence figures are exceedingly difficult to interpret and use operationally in a meaningful way.

There are three main reasons for this:

- prevalence rates are likely to fluctuate over time by 5% which impedes the accurate description of trends;
- prevalence rates do not readily capture information on non-hospital acquired pressure sores;
- prevalence data do not describe the duration of the pressure sores.

However, several authors have described difficulty in undertaking the process of incidence monitoring (Clark and Watts, 1994; Molyneux, 1994), indicating that the effort required to undertake this initiative should not be underestimated.

## Areas to be Included in Audit

The demographic characteristics of the patient population being audited should be known. The inclusion or exclusion of low-risk patient groups such as those receiving maternity or paediatric services will have a profound effect on aggregate prevalence rates.

## Classification of Pressure Sores

It is stated very strongly in the literature that the lack of consistency in the classification of skin pressure damage makes it difficult to compare the results of many published pressure sore incidence/prevalence surveys. Lack of uniformity of grading occurs frequently at the lower end of the scale of pressure damage, with some authors failing to identify non-blanching erythema as pressure damage (O'Dea, 1993).

Non-blanching erythema (a term used to descri⌐ that has reddened and which does not whiten wher sure is applied) is considered to represent the fi⌐ pressure damage (Ribbe and Van Marum, 1993).

The Department of Health publication (1993ᴅ) ... A Key Quality Indicator' describes the following classification scheme which is a form of the UK Consensus Classification of Pressure Sore Severity, as reported by Reid and Morison (1994):

Stage 1    Discolorations of intact skin, including non-blanchable erythema, and blue/purple and black discoloration.

Stage 2    Partial thickness skin loss or damage involving the epidermis and/or dermis.

Stage 3    Full-thickness skin loss involving damage or necrosis of subcutaneous tissues, but not through the underlying fascia and not extending to the underlying bone, tendon or joint capsule.

Stage 4    Full-thickness skin loss with extensive destruction and tissue necrosis extending to the underlying bone, tendon or joint capsule.

An additional consideration in relation to the classification of pressure sores is whether or not sores are hospital acquired or otherwise. Richardson (1993) reported that, during 1991, 28% of pressure sores were present on admission to a large general hospital (total number of patients 1021). The segregation of hospital acquired versus non-hospital acquired pressure sore incidence rates enables a more accurate description of the nature and extent of the pressure sore problem within a hospital.

## Methods of Data Collection

In-house prevalence surveys require auditors to undertake training sessions to ensure that a common approach to data collection exists, which is characterised by high rater-reliability. In addition pro-forma data collection sheets need to be designed. Alternatively external agencies, such as pressure-relieving equipment hire companies, will undertake prevalence surveys.

Incidence surveillance requires the development of pro-forma data collection sheets and a system for the storage and retrieval of these data sheets (for example, Figure 11.1).

**CHELSEA & WESTMINSTER HEALTHCARE NHS TRUST**

PRESSURE SORE INCIDENCE MONITORING FORM

Ward ..................

Completed for the period from week commencing Monday ............. (insert date) to Sunday ............ (insert date).
Please give details of all patients who have a pressure sore. This will include those patients who have discolouration of intact skin (grade 1 pressure sore - see overleaf for classification scheme).

| Patient details<br>*Please provide patient name and hospital number* | Date admitted to ward | Source of admission<br>*For example, another ward, another hospital, home etc.* | Date pressure sore(s) first observed | Grade of pressure sore(s)<br>*Please use the classification scheme printed overleaf.* | Location of pressure sore(s)<br>*For example, sacrum, left buttock, right elbow etc.* | Specific nursing care interventions<br>*For example, dietary supplements, pressure relieving bed / chair devices, positioning / mobilisation regime etc.* | Pressure sore risk assessment score<br>*Please indicate the risk assessment tool employed, for example Waterlow, Braden, PSPS etc.* |
|---|---|---|---|---|---|---|---|
| | | | | | | | |
| | | | | | | | |
| | | | | | | | |

Completed by ................. (please give signature, name in print and designation).

**Figure 11.1** Example of a Pressure Sore Incidence Monitoring Form as used at Chelsea & Westminster Hospital, London

The need for any incidence monitoring system to be managed or overseen by a named individual is identified by several authors as important in ensuring that full participation with the initiative occurs (for example, Molyneux, 1994).

## Data Analysis

An appropriate agency for the analysis and presentation of data, such as a clinical audit department, should be identified prior to the onset of the audit process.

## Data Reporting

Who presents the data and in what format should also be predetermined. It may be considered appropriate that whilst information pertaining to the individual directorates is widely available, information pertaining to individual wards is not generally available throughout the organisation. Molyneux (1994) describes how providing staff with timely feedback relating to the occurrence of pressure sores in their ward/department was an important factor in motivating them to be consistent and careful in their pressure sore incidence monitoring.

## Standard of Care: Prevention of Pressure Sores

(as employed in Chelsea & Westminster Healthcare NHS Trust)

*Outcome criteria*

1.  All healthcare professionals will have the research-based knowledge required to manage patients who are at risk of developing pressure sores as identified in the pressure sore prevention strategy document.
2.  Resources required for the prevention of pressure sores will be deployed in an effective way, according to patient needs in each clinical area.
3.  Patients will have the information which they require in order to contribute to planned pressure sore prevention care and treatment.
4.  There will be evidence of a full and up-to-date record for each patient, detailing:

Assessment of pressure sore risk
Planned care appropriate to the patient's risk of developing pressure sores
Care interventions
Evaluation of the outcomes of care interventions.

5.   Pressure sore incidence/prevalence will reduce in each clinical area.

*Structure criteria*

1.   There will be a copy of the pressure sore prevention strategy document in all clinical areas and accessible to all staff.
2.   All healthcare professionals will have access to training and education in relation to pressure sore prevention.
3.   Staff will possess knowledge and understanding in relation to pressure sore risk assessment, i.e. the predisposing and precipitating factors involved.
4.   Staff will possess knowledge of care and treatment interventions appropriate to a patient's risk of developing pressure sores.
5.   Information on equipment ordering procedures will be available at ward level.
6.   Pressure sore prevention equipment, together with information about its use and maintenance, will be readily available.
7.   Resources required for effective pressure sore prevention will be provided at a level which meets service demand.
8.   All staff will receive training in relation to patient lifting and handling techniques each year.
9.   Every clinical area will have written information about pressure sore prevention available to their patients.
10.  Each member of the multidisciplinary team will be aware of the roles of colleagues in pressure sore prevention, and seek advice from appropriate sources as necessary.
11.  Each member of the multidisciplinary team will be responsible for maintaining and updating his or her knowledge in relation to pressure sore prevention.

*Process criteria*

1.   Within 1 hour of admission to hospital all patients will be assessed by a Registered Nurse for risk of pressure sore development, and this will be recorded in their nursing notes within 12 hours of admission to hospital.

2.  Risk of pressure sore development will be assessed using professional judgement, with consideration for known predisposing and precipitating factors, and by using an appropriate risk assessment tool to aid this process.

3.  Internal audit of inter-rater reliability of using the risk assessment tool employed will be conducted every 3 months to assess whether scores are being similarly assigned.

4.  Communication of a patient's risk of pressure sore development, and any care initiated in relation to this risk, will occur between all departments and multidisciplinary team members involved in a patient's care or treatment.

5.  Pressure-relieving equipment, appropriate to the patient's risk of developing pressure sores, will be installed within 4 hours of admission to hospital.

6.  An individual pressure sore prevention plan of care will be developed within 12 hours of admission to hospital, with consideration of identified predisposing and precipitating risk factors.

7.  Care planned will be congruent with research findings, as indicated in the pressure sore prevention strategy.

8.  Evaluation of the outcomes of care interventions will occur at least weekly, with evidence of a subsequent review of care planned as appropriate.

9.  Reassessment of a patient's risk of developing pressure sores will occur at least weekly and whenever there is any change of condition, intervention, e.g. surgery, or changes to the patient's daily activities of living.

10. Each clinical area should give consideration to the special needs of its patient group and appropriately develop a local strategy for the prevention of pressure sores.

11. All clinical areas will collect pressure sore incidence data weekly; the data are to be used for:
    Evaluation of pressure sore prevention strategies
    Evaluation of effectiveness of resource deployment
    Identification of training/education needs of staff.

12. At least once every 5 years, each member of staff should attend a study day on the prevention of pressure sores.

# Standard of Care: Mattress Replacement

(as employed in Chelsea & Westminster Healthcare NHS Trust)

*Outcome criteria*

1.  All patients will be provided with a mattress which conforms to Department of Health standards, and which is comfortable and hygienic.
2.  Mattresses will be maintained in a condition which is acceptable, or replaced if unsatisfactory.
3.  A mattress replacement programme will operate in each clinical area.

*Structure criteria*

1.  A designated member of staff will be responsible for auditing mattresses in his or her clinical area.
2.  The designated staff member will have knowledge of mattress audit methods, in line with the recommended audit tool provided.
3.  Each clinical area will develop a mattress replacement strategy.

*Process criteria*

1.  Mattresses will be dated at the time of their issue to the wards.
2.  A mattress-turning regimen will be employed by each clinical area.
3.  A mattress-cleaning policy, which is congruent with infection control policy and manufacturers' recommendations, will be employed consistently by each clinical area.
4.  An audit of mattress condition will be conducted every 6 months by the designated staff member in each clinical area using the tool provided.

# References

Anthony D (1987) Pointers to good care. Nursing Times 83(34): 27–30.

Audit Commission (1991) The Virtue of Patients: Making the Best Use of Ward Nursing Resources. London: The Audit Commission for Local Authorities and the National Health Service.

Bader DL (Ed) (1990) Pressure Sores: Clinical Practice and Scientific Approach. London: Macmillan Press.

Bader DL, Gant CA (1988) Changes in transcutaneous oxygen tension as a result of prolonged pressures at the sacrum. Clinical Physiological Measurement 9: 33–40.

Baird RM (1979) Microbial contamination of topical medications used in treatment and prevention of pressure sores. Journal of Hygiene. Cited in Torrance C (1983) Pressure Sores: Aetiology, Treatment and Prevention. London: Croom Helm.

Bar CA (1991) Evaluation of cushions using dynamic pressure measurement. Prosthetics and Orthotics International 15: 245–51. Cited in Vohra RK, McCollum CN (1994) Pressure sores. British Medical Journal 309: 853–7.

Barbenal JC, Jordan MM, Nichol SM, Clark MO (1977) Incidence of pressure sores in the Greater Glasgow Health Board area. Lancet 2: 548–50.

Barton A (1977) Prevention of pressure sores. Nursing Times 73(41): 1593–5.

Berecek KH (1975) Treatment of decubitus ulcers. Nursing Clinics of North America 10(1): 171–210. Cited in Torrance C (1983) Pressure Sores: Aetiology, Treatment and Prevention: London: Croom Helm.

Bergstrom N, Braden BJ, Laguzza A et al. (1987) The Braden scale for predicting pressure sore risk. Nursing Research 36(4): 205–10.

Berlowitz DR (1989) Risk factors for pressure sores: a comparison of cross-sectional and cohort derived data. Journal of the American Geriatrics Society 37: 1043–50.

Bliss MR (1988) Prevention and management of pressure sores. Update 1 May (36): 2258–67.

Bliss MR, Thomas JM (1993) Making sense of comparative values. Evaluation of constant low pressure supports. Professional Nurse 8(9): 564–70.

Braden BJ, Bergstrom N (1989) Clinical utility of the Braden scale for predicting pressure risk. Decubitus 2(3): 44–51.

Brand PW (1976) Pressure sores — the problem. In Kenedi RM, Cowden JM, Scales JT Bed Sore Biomechanics. Baltimore: University Park Press. pp 19–23.

Breslow RA (1993) The importance of dietary protein in healing pressure ulcers. Journal of the American Geriatrics Society 41(4): 357–62.

Bridel J (1993) Assessing the risk of pressure sores. Nursing Standard 7(25): 32–5.

Bridel J (1994) Risk assessment. Journal of Tissue Viability 4(3): 84–5.

Chapman EJ, Chapman R (1986) Treatment of pressure sores: the state of the art. In Tierney A (Ed) Clinical Nursing Practice. Edinburgh: Churchill Livingstone.

Clark M, Watts S (1994) The incidence of pressure sores within a National Health Service Trust during 1991. Journal of Advanced Nursing 20(1): 33–6.

Cohen C (1968) Zinc sulphate and bedsores. British Medical Journal 2: 561.

Cullum N, Shakespeare P (1994) Pressure sores — a key quality indicator. Journal of Tissue Viability 4(2): 60–1.

David JA, Chapman RG, Chapman EJ and Lockett B (1983) An Investigation of the Current Methods used in Nursing for the Care of Patients with Established Pressure Sores. Nursing Practice Research Unit, Northwick Park Hospital and Clinical Research Centre.

David J (1987) Wound Management. London: Martin Dunitz.

Davies K, Strickland J, Laurence V, Duncan A and Rowe J (1991) The hidden mortality from pressure sores. Journal of Tissue Viability 1(18).

Dealey C (1989) Risk assessment of pressure sores. A comparative study of the Norton and Waterlow scores. CARE — Science & Practice 7(1): 5–7.

Dealey C (1991) The size of the pressure sore problem in a teaching hospital. Journal of Advanced Nursing 16(6): 663–70.

Dealey C (1992a) Pressure sores — the result of bad nursing? British Journal of Nursing 1(15): 748.

Dealey C (1992b) Specific hospital problems in the prevention and management of pressure sores. Journal of Tissue Viability 2(4) 36–7.

Department of Health (1992) The Health of the Nation: A Strategy for Health in England. London: HMSO.

Department of Health (1993a) Pressure Sores: A Key Quality Indicator. Department of Health. London: Health Publications Unit.

Department of Health (1993b) Foam Mattresses: A Comparative Evaluation. Evaluation PS1. Medical Devices Directorate. London: HMSO.

Department of Health (1994) Static Mattress Overlays — A Comparative Evaluation. Evaluation PS2. Medical Devices Directorate. London: HMSO.

Dimond B (1994) Pressure sores: a case to answer. British Journal of Nursing 3(14): 721–7.

Dinsdale SM (1973) Decubitus ulcers in swine: light and electron microscope study of pathogenesis. Archives of Physical Medicine and Rehabilitation 54: 51–6. Cited in Torrance C (1983) Pressure Sores: Aetiology, Treatment and Prevention. London: Croom Helm.

Dyson R (1978) Bedsores — the injuries hospital staff inflict on patients. Nursing Mirror 146(24): 30–2.

Edwards M (1994) The rationale for the use of risk calculators in pressure sore prevention, and evidence of the reliability and validity of published scales. Journal of Advanced Nursing 22: 288–96.

Exton-Smith AN (1961) The prevention of pressure sores: the significance of spontaneous bodily movements. Lancet 2: 1124–6. Cited in Malone C (1992) Intensive pressures. Nursing Times 88(36): 57–62.

Flanagan M (1993) Pressure sore risk assessment scales. Journal of Wound Care 2(3): 162–7.

Gebhardt K, Bliss MR (1994) Preventing pressure sores in orthopaedic patients — is prolonged chair nursing detrimental? Journal of Tissue Viability 4(2): 51–4.

Goode HF, Burns E and Walker BE (1992) Vitamin C depletion and pressure sores in elderly patients with femoral neck fracture. British Medical Journal 305: 925–7.

Groth KE (1942) Clinical observations and experimental studies on the origin of decubiti. Acta Chirurgica Scandinavica 87 (Supplement 76): 1–209. Cited in Kelly J (1994) The aetiology of pressure sores. Journal of Tissue Viability 4(3): 77–8.

Hibbs P (1988) Action against pressure sores. Nursing Times 84(13): 68–73.

Hill L (1992) The question of pressure. Nursing Times 88(12): 76–82.

Johnson J (1994) Pressure area risk assessment in a neurological setting. British Journal of Nursing 3(18): 926–35.

Kelly J (1994) The aetiology of pressure sores. Journal of Tissue Viability 4(3): 77.

Kenedi RM, Cowden JM (Eds) (1975) Bed sore diomechanics: proceedings of a seminar an tissue viability and clinical applications held at the University of Strathclyde Glasgow; Glasgow; University of Strathclyde Bioengineering Department.

Khanh (1984) An in-depth look at pressure sores using monolithic silicon pressure sensors. Plastic and Reconstructive Surgery December: 745–54.

King's Fund Centre (1989) The Prevention and Management of Pressure Sores within Health Districts. London: King's Fund Centre for Health Services Development.

Kosiak M (1959) Etiology and pathology of decubitus ulcers. Archives of Physical Medicine and Rehabilitation 40: 62–9. Cited in Vohra RK, McCollum CN (1994) Pressure sores. British Medical Journal 309: 853–7.

Landis EM (1930) Micro-injection studies of capillary blood pressure in human skin. Heart 15: 209–28. Cited in Burman PMS (1994) Measuring pressure. Journal of Wound Care 3(2): 83–6.

Larsson J (1990) Effect of dietary supplement on nutritional status and clinical outcome in 501 geriatric patients — a randomised study. Clinical Nutrition 9: 179–84.

Lennard-Jones JE (1992) A Positive Approach to Nutrition as Treatment. London: King's Fund Centre for Health Services Development.

Lincoln R et al (1986) Use of the Nortan pressure sore risk assessment scoring system with elderly patients in an acute area. Journal of Esterostomal Therapy 15(5): 201–5.

Livesley B (1987) Pressure sores: an expensive epidemic. Nursing Times 83(6): 79.

Livesley B (1990) Pressure sores: clinical aspects of their cost, causation and prevention. Cited in Bader DL, (Ed) (1990) Pressure Sores — Clinical Practice and Scientific Approach. London: Macmillan Press.

Lockyer-Stevens N (1993) The use of water-filled gloves to prevent the formation of decubitus ulcers on heels. Journal of Wound Care 2(4): 282–5.

Lockyer-Stevens N (1994) Methods for auditing pressure sores. Nursing Standard 8(34): 60–2.

Lowry M (1992) Hospital seating and pressure areas. Nursing Standard 6(34): 10–12.

Lowthian P (1979) Turning clocks system to prevent pressure sores. Nursing Mirror 148(21): 10–31. Cited in Torrance C (1983) Pressure Sores: Aetiology, Treatment and Prevention. London: Croom Helm.

Lowthian P (1982) Review of pressure sore pathogenesis. Nursing Times 78(3): 117–9.

Lowthian P (1987) Classification and grading of pressure sores. CARE — Science & Practice 5(1): 5–9.

Lowthian P (1993) Acute patient care: Pressure areas. British Journal of Nursing 2(9): 449–50.

Lowthian P (1994) Letter to the editor. Journal of Tissue Viability 4(2): 62.

Marchand AC, Lidowski H (1993) Reassessment of the use of genuine sheepskin for pressure ulcer prevention and treatment. Decubitus 6(1): 44–7.

McTaggart J (1994) An area of clinical neglect — evaluation of healing status in wound care. Professional Nurse 9(9): 600–6.

Michel CC (1990) Microvascular mechanisms in stasis ischaemia. Cited in Bader DL (Ed) (1990) Pressure Sores — Clinical Practice and Scientific Approach. London: Macmillan Press.

Middleton D (1983) Nursing. Oxford: Blackwell Scientific Publications.

Molyneux R (1994) Pressure sore surveillance — evolution of a system in one health district. Journal of Tissue Viability 4(2): 56–9.

Moolton WP (1972) Bedsores in the chronically ill patient. Archives of Physical Medicine and Rehabilitation 53: 430–80. Cited in Torrance C (1983) Pressure Sores: Aetiology, Treatment and Prevention. London: Croom Helm.

Norton D (1962) An Investigation of Geriatric Nursing Problems in Hospital. London: National Corporation for the Care of Old People.

Norton D (1989) Calculating the risk: reflections on the Norton scale. Decubitus 2(3): 24–31.

Norton D et al. (1962) An investigation of geriatric nursing problems in hospitals. London: Corporation for the Care of Old People. Cited in Vohra RK, McCollum CN (1994) Pressure sores. British Medical Journal 309: 853–7.

O'Dea K (1993) Prevalence of pressure damage in hospital patients in the UK. Journal of Wound Care 2(4): 221–5.

Oswald J, Adam K (1984) Sleep helps healing. British Medical Journal 289: 1400–1.

Preston KW (1988) Positioning for comfort and pressure relief: the 30 degree alternative. CARE — Science & Practice 6(4): 116–9.

Pritchard AP, David JA (1984) The Royal Marsden Hospital Manual of Clinical Nursing Procedures. London: Harper & Row.

Pritchard V |(1986) Pressure Sores Supplement. Calculating the risk. Nursing Times 82: 59–61.

Reid J, Morison M (1994) Towards consensus: classification of pressure sores. Journal of Wound Care 3(3) 157–60.

Reswick JB, Rogers J (1976) Experience at Ranchos Los Amigos Hospital with devices and techniques to prevent pressure sores. Cited in Kennedi RM, Cowden JM, Scales JT (1976) Bedsore Biomechanics. Baltimore: University Park Press. 301–13.

Reuler IB, Cooney TJ (1981) The pressure sore: pathophysiology and principles of management. Annals of Internal Medicine 94: 661–6.

Ribbe MW, Van Marum RJ (1993) Decubitus; pathophysiology clinical symptoms and susceptibility. Journal of Tissue Viability 2(4): 119–20.

Richardson B (1993) Hospital versus community acquired pressure sores: Should prevalence rates be separated. Journal of Tissue Viability 3(1): 13–15.

Rithalia S (1993) Reducing the pressure. Nursing Times 89(42): 67–8.

Robertson JC (1987) £100,000 damages for a pressure sore. CARE — Science & Practice 5(2).

Royal College of Nursing (1993) The Role of the Support Worker within the Professional Nursing Team. London: Royal College of Nursing.

Salvadalena G, Snyder M, Brogdon K (1992) Clinical trial of the Braden scale on an acute medical care unit. Journal of E.T. Nursing 19: 160–5.

Schubert V, Fagrell B (1989) Local skin pressure and its effects on skin microsectional and cohort derived data. Journal of the American Geriatrics Society 37: 1043–50.

Shakespeare P (1994) Scoring the risk score. Journal of Tissue Viability 4(1): 21–2.

Staas WE, Cioschi HM (1991) Pressure sores: a multifaceted approach to prevention and treatment. Western Journal of Medicine 154: 539–44. Cited in Vohra RK, McCollum CN (1994) Pressure sores. British Medical Journal 309: 853–7.

Sutton JC, Wallace WA (1990) Pressure sores: the views and practices of senior hospital doctors. Clinical Rehabilitation 4: 137–43.

Torrance C (1983) Pressure Sores: Aetiology, Treatment and Prevention. London: Croom Helm.

Tuttle SG (1965) Further observations on amino acid requirements of older men. American Journal of Clinical Nutrition 16(2): 225–31. Cited in Torrance C (1983) Pressure Sores: Aetiology, Treatment and Prevention. London: Croom Helm.

UKCC (1992) Code of Professional Conduct. 3rd edn. London: UKCC.

UKCC (1993) Standards for Records and Record Keeping. London: UKCC.

Vasile J, Chaitin H (1972) Prognostic factors in decubitus ulcers of the aged. Geriatrics 27: 126–9. Cited in Torrance C (1983) Pressure Sores: Aetiology, Treatment and Prevention. London: Croom Helm.

Vohra RK, McCollum CN (1994) Pressure sores. British Journal of Medicine 309: 853–7.

Waterlow J (1987) Calculating the risk. Nursing Times 83(39): 58–60.

Waterlow J (1988a) The Waterlow card for prevention and management of pressure sores: towards a pocket policy. CARE — Science & Practice 6(1): 8–12.

Waterlow J (1988b) Prevention is cheaper than cure. Nursing Times 84(25): 69–70.

Waterlow J (1991) A policy that protects. The Waterlow pressure sore prevention/treatment policy. Professional Nurse 6(5): 258, 260, 262–4.

Waterlow J (1995) Pressure Sore Prevention Manual. (Available from Mrs J Waterlow, Newtons, Curland, Taunton TA3 3SG, UK. Price £2.50. Copies of the Waterlow Card are available price 22p each.)

Whimster I (1976) Bedsore Biomechanics. London: Macmillan Press.

Williams C (1992) A comparative study of pressure sore prevention scores. Journal of Tissue Viability 2(2): 64–6.

Wilson M (1985) Surgical Nursing 11th edn. London: Bailliere Tindall.

Young J (1990) Preventing pressure sores: Does the mattress work? Journal of Tissue Viability 2(1): 17.

Young JB, Dobrzanski S (1992) Pressure sores: epidemiology and current management concepts. Drugs and Ageing 2(1): 42–57.

# Index